The Pandemic Crisis and the European Union

This book assesses the implications of the COVID-19 pandemic for the European Union (EU), as well as its response in dealing with an overarching, multidimensional crisis with consequences extending beyond public health safety to political, economic, legal and institutional arenas.

It argues the pandemic represents a symmetric crisis cutting across countries with different social, economic and political characteristics and which yet – despite favouring cooperative solutions at the supranational level – has largely been met with initial responses of a national, even local, nature. So, how well did the EU perform as a crisis manager in the pandemic crisis?

This book will be of key interest to scholars, students and readers of crisis, pandemic and health management, European Union politics and governance.

Paulo Vila Maior is Associate Professor of European Studies at the University Fernando Pessoa and Researcher at CEPESE, Porto, Portugal.

Isabel Camisão is Assistant Professor in European Studies at the University of Coimbra, and Researcher at CICP, Braga and Évora, Portugal.

Routledge Advances in European Politics

Changing Perceptions of the EU at Times of Brexit
Global perspectives
Edited by Natalia Chaban, Arne Niemann and Johanna Speyer

The EU through Multiple Crises
Representation and cohesion dilemmas for a "sui generis" polity
Edited by Maurizio Cotta and Pierangelo Isernia

Linguistic Claims and Political Conflicts
Spanish labyrinths in the European Context
Andrea C. Bianculli, Jacint Jordana and Mónica Ferrín Pereira

EU–Korea Security Relations
Edited by Nicola Casarini

European Futures
Challenges and crossroads for the European Union of 2050
Edited by Chad Damro, Elke Heins and Drew Scott

Poland and Germany in the European Union
The multi-dimensional dynamics of bilateral relations
Edited by Elżbieta Opiłowska and Monika Sus

Electoral Politics in Crisis After the Great Recession
Change, fluctuations and stability in Iceland
Eva H. Önnudóttir, Agnar Freyr Helgason, Olafur Th. Hardarson and Hulda Thórisdóttir

The Pandemic Crisis and the European Union
COVID-19 and crisis management
Paulo Vila Maior and Isabel Camisão

For more information about this series, please visit: www.routledge.com/Routledge-Advances-in-European-Politics/book-series/AEP

The Pandemic Crisis and the European Union

COVID-19 and Crisis Management

Paulo Vila Maior and Isabel Camisão

Routledge
Taylor & Francis Group
LONDON AND NEW YORK

First published 2022
by Routledge
2 Park Square, Milton Park, Abingdon, Oxon OX14 4RN

and by Routledge
605 Third Avenue, New York, NY 10158

Routledge is an imprint of the Taylor & Francis Group, an informa business

British Library Cataloguing-in-Publication Data
A catalogue record for this book is available from the British Library

Library of Congress Cataloging-in-Publication Data
Names: Vila Maior, Paulo, author. | Camisão, Isabel, author.
Title: The pandemic crisis and the European Union: COVID-19 and crisis management / Paulo Vila Maior and Isabel Camisão.
Description: Abingdon, Oxon; New York, NY: Routledge, 2022. |
Series: Routledge advances in European politics |
Includes bibliographical references and index.
Identifiers: LCCN 2021022403 (print) | LCCN 2021022404 (ebook) |
ISBN 9780367722081 (hardback) | ISBN 9780367722135 (paperback) |
ISBN 9781003153900 (ebook)
Subjects: LCSH: Public health–European Union countries. |
Medical policy–European Union countries. |
COVID-19 (Disease)–Economic aspects. | COVID-19 (Disease)–Social aspects.
Classification: LCC RA483 .V55 2022 (print) | LCC RA483 (ebook) |
DDC 362.1962/4140094–dc23
LC record available at https://lccn.loc.gov/2021022403
LC ebook record available at https://lccn.loc.gov/2021022404

ISBN: 978-0-367-72208-1 (hbk)
ISBN: 978-0-367-72213-5 (pbk)
ISBN: 978-1-003-15390-0 (ebk)

DOI: 10.4324/9781003153900

Typeset in Times New Roman
by Newgen Publishing UK

Contents

Illustrations

Figures

Tables

Acknowledgements

This study was conducted at Research Center in Political Science (UID/CPO/0758/2019), University of Minho/University of Évora and supported by the Portuguese Foundation for Science and Technology and the Portuguese Ministry of Education and Science through national funds.

FCT Fundação para a Ciência e a Tecnologia

cicp Centro de Investigação em Ciência Política

Abbreviations

CAA	Crisis Coordination Arrangements
CEAS	Common European Asylum System
CRII	Corona Response Investment Initiative
CRT	Corona Response Team
ECB	European Central Bank
ECDC	European Centre for Disease Prevention and Control
ECJ	European Court of Justice
ECSC	European Coal and Steel Community
EEC	European Economic Community
EES	Entry/Exit System
EMA	European Medicines Agency
EMU	Economic and Monetary Union
EP	European Parliament
EPSCO	Employment, Social Policy, Health and Consumer Affairs
ERCC	Emergency Response Coordination Centre
ETIAS	European Traveller Information and Authorisation System
EU	European Union
EWRS	Early Warning and Response System
GDP	Gross Domestic Product
HERA	Health Emergency Response Authority
HSC	Heath Security Committee
IPCR	Integrated Political Crisis Response
IR	International Relations
JPA	Joint Procurement Agreement
MFF	Multiannual Financial Framework
OMT	Outright Monetary Transactions
PEPP	Pandemic Emergency Purchase Programme
PPE	Personal Protective Equipment
REACT-EU	Recovery Assistance for Cohesion and the Territories of Europe
SARS	Severe Acute Respiratory Syndrome
SBC	Schengen Borders Code
SGP	Stability and Growth Pact

SIS	Schengen Information System
TEU	Treaty on the European Union
TFEU	Treaty on the Functioning of the European Union
US	United States
WHO	World Health Organisation

Introduction

COVID-19 and the European Union – is this time really for bad?

I.1 Introduction

On 24 January 2020 the first case of COVID-19 was reported within the European Union (EU). At that time, Europe, and the rest of the world, were far from anticipating the true dimension of the crisis that was forming. COVID-19 pandemic is a transversal crisis, cutting across countries with different social, economic and political characteristics, wealthier and developing countries all together. For its highly contagious potential, COVID-19 forced authorities around the globe to enforce legal measures that implemented lockdown to variable degrees, which eventually paralysed a large part of member states' economic activities. At some point, the world was forcefully brought to a halt. Companies were shut down, bringing massive amounts of workers to layoff or to unemployment. Production and consumption hit historical lows. As households' income decreased, the economy further slowed down, paving the way for deep worldwide recession.[1]

A world characterised by unique patterns of globalisation and interdependence resorted to national, not to mention local, solutions and unilateral remedies. In extreme cases, lockdown forced persons to stay in their municipality, with no contact with neighbouring villages. Governments realised that macroeconomic plans ought to be revised, as the sudden change of circumstances implied a different sort of challenges for economic policy. Before economic indicators started to show the true dimension of the economic crisis, a profound impact on countries' macroeconomic performance was grounded on the unprecedented effects of the (at the time) would-be crisis triggered by the proliferation of the pandemic.

In Europe, mechanisms of European integration were again brought to the fore. Established patters of governance in the EU draw attention to solutions at the supranational level. The explanation is twofold. On the one hand, since the pandemic faces no borders and all member states are affected to variable degrees, it was expected that a coordinated effort at the EU level was the appropriate answer to immediate challenges stemming from the spread of the virus. On the other hand, the medium-term effects of the ensuing crisis, centred on the political-economic arena, cannot not be disregarded. Expected

DOI: 10.4324/9781003153900-1

macroeconomic implications resulting from measures to contain the pandemic are difficult to revert.

I.2 Rationale of the book

COVID-19 is a critical juncture[2] for the EU, for the aforementioned reasons. It was not by accident that, as Angela Merkel put it bluntly, this was the biggest challenge Europe faced since the European Communities were created.[3] Despite the fact that crisis is a genetic imprint of European integration, crisis is never démodé in the EU and its member states. It encompasses a meaning that goes beyond the conventional understanding of crisis as bearing an economic watermark. Its manifold dimensions include social, political, institutional, constitutional, cultural, even philosophical aspects that act on their own or intertwine in different combinations, in different moments and in different places. Another layer of complexity is added by recognising that the combination of different parcels of the crisis is prone to subjectivism. The pandemic crisis is another layer added to the permanent sense of crisis that hangs over citizens, politicians, analysts, social scientists and others. Indeed, the EU has been muddling through different instances of crises, sometimes crises within crisis (like a palimpsest of crises), as if crises were the engines of (more) Europe. The rationale is well documented on several analyses of European integration history.

The initial perception was that 'this time is for bad,' not only for the potentially catastrophic, multidimensional effects of the pandemic, but also because (differently from previous crisis) this is a symmetric crisis. We use this expression as a purposeful debasement of the long-established, mainstream expression 'this time is for good.' When people warrant 'this time is for good,' an inescapable opportunity for change is implied. That is precisely the challenge that stems from the pandemic, as we argue. Nevertheless, we decided to adjust the expression to accommodate the expectable damaging effects of a misadjusted or late response to the pandemic crisis on the social, political, economic, legal and institutional arenas. The challenge goes well beyond the public health response encompassing a multidimensional nature: for citizens at large (maybe, altered ways of living in the aftermath of the pandemic); for decision-makers, particularly economic policy decision-makers (the design of the appropriate economic policy mix when medium-term implications of short-term economic policy measures that address immediate social-economic effects of the pandemic crisis are at stake); for constitutionalists and legal experts in general (facing the future implications of exceptional measures designed to mitigate the propagation of the virus, notably to what extent exceptionalism paves the road for a new rule); and for the EU as a polity, in the face of the institutional dynamics during the (not so much, not always) coordinated reaction to the pandemic and to the following economic and social crisis.

Hence, by 'this time is for bad' we mean it is 'now or never' (if the deterministic overemphasis is discounted by the reader). Prospects also bear an unprecedented imprint. This is a symmetric crisis (with minor nuances, when it comes to assess to what extent member states were impacted by the pandemic), putting national governments in the same playing field. What is more, the effects of the pandemic and the correlated crisis bring to the surface a truly existential threat to the EU should it not be able (or willing) to provide joint action to respond to this unparalleled challenge.

The book focuses on the implications of the pandemic for the EU. Despite the EU being centripetal to this analysis, we are aware that it cannot be disentangled from participating countries. Although it is an actor on its own, the EU is prone to influences exerted by member states. On the one hand, representatives of national governments have a seat in two influential institutions of the EU (the European Council and the Council of the European Union). The former provides political guidelines to European integration and a broad sense of political leadership. The latter is a key actor on the EU's decision-making dynamics, as it participates in negotiations with the European Parliament (EP) concerning legislative proposals submitted by the European Commission. On the other hand, notwithstanding institutional independence of other important institutions of the EU (the EP, the European Commission and the European Central Bank (ECB), just to mention political institutions), with the implication that they are not permeable to national interests, this is not always the case. Members of the EP are accountable to their European political groups but are also frequently sensible to national interests of the member state of their nationality. The embeddedness of the European Commission's activity with national interests is more nuanced and difficult to demonstrate, since the overall perception is that commissioners are able to act independently from other institutions and, crucially, from national interests of the national government that appointed him/her. The same remark holds as far as the ECB is considered, notably for the six members of the Executive Committee, on grounds of the extensive status of political independence granted to the monetary authority. These are the institutions of the EU that count for our analysis regarding the effects of the pandemic crisis at the level of EU institutions.

Yet, national governments possess many channels to wield influence on the EU decision-making process and politics in general. This aspect is important for the scope of the book. Whereas attention is paid on discussions, recommendations, legal acts and political orientations at the level of EU institutions, the national level is not left outside the analysis. This does not mean that national governments' particular reactions to the pandemic will be addressed. That is not the reach of the book. Since national governments interact within the institutional system of the EU, their positions, their claims and their arguments will also rank high among the priorities of the book. In addition, it is, to a large extent, countries' positions, their proactive stance or inertia, that give ground to fundamental inputs for the EU as an actor on the pandemic. A sample of some national governments' decisions on the sanitary dimension of the crisis, as well as some national governments' reported influence in EU institutions, will be accounted for.

Change (along with crisis) is the operational concept that cuts across the book's analysis. We measure change using a comparative lens where relevant actors' leverage is taken in consideration. COVID-19 is the hallmark for the comparative exercise, by taking stock of the influence exerted by actors in the pre- and post-COVID-19 scenarios. The context prior to the pandemic is well documented: how did actors interact and to what extent were they influential in the policy areas that match with the several dimensions of the pandemic crisis outlined in the following chapters. The challenge is to find out whether continuity or discontinuity characterises the institutional system by looking at the way actors were able to influence relevant decisions to address the crisis. In this exercise, we ask whether institutional re-balancing of some sort is one implication of the pandemic crisis.

The book follows a holistic approach to COVID-19 crisis in tune with the multidimensionality of the crisis. Short-term answers stemming from the fight against the pandemic involve political answers at the level of economic policy, social policy, humanitarian action, market regulation, security issues and the awareness of how emergency asks for constitutional exceptionality. Accordingly, the book takes a comprehensive approach that incorporates all these dimensions into the analytical framework.

I.3 Structure of the book

Chapter 1 unveils the theoretical framework of the book. Pegging on the notions of perennial crisis (Nanopoulos and Vergis, 2019) and of 'slow-burning' crisis (Boin, Ekengren and Rhinard, 2020) we look to previous crises that affected the EU and its member states and draw a comparison to find out similarities and dissimilarities between these crises and the pandemic crisis. We will also look for patterns of continuity or discontinuity both in the processes and results' dimensions. The potential for change is assessed using Streeck and Thelen's model (2005) for analysing institutional change.

The theoretical framework anchors the perception that crises have been a driving force of European integration, as if they provided the opportunity for a leap forward. Crises are not limited to economic crisis, maybe the most obvious contender when the analysis of crises in the EU is at stake. They are multidimensional and enmesh with each other at a randomised scale. In addition to economic crisis, other examples place the EU within a perpetual scenario where social, political, institutional, legal, cultural and even philosophical crises intertwine.

The play is variable over time and within the manifold dimensions of the crisis. The pattern is also not constant over time. Throughout the history of European integration, several episodes of crises played out. They did not affect member states consistently, as not all countries were disturbed, and some were struck more violently than others. What matters for Chapter 1 is to recognise that continuing crisis was a sanctuary of European integration, as in many cases solutions devised at the supranational level were the panacea for the problems at stake. To a certain extent, we resort to a utilitarian-based approach of European integration, cogent with Milward's analysis (1999) that envisages the European Communities (and later the EU) as a scapegoat for nation-states' reaction to the vagaries of increased globalisation and interdependence. National governments learned to accommodate to the EU as a regime, with an institutional system of its own and a delimitation of competences between the EU and member states, bestowing the recognition of how centripetal the EU has been to address (but not always to solve) many episodes of crisis that hindered member states in the first place.

In Chapter 1 we follow the narrative of 'this time is for bad' to argue that important divergences prevent the pandemic from a linear comparison with previous crises. Above all, the symmetry of the pandemic crisis is the evidence of substantial differences. While in the past crises were, one way or the other, asymmetric in nature, the pandemic affected all member states. Even though there are some differences in terms of the severity of public health effects – some member states were stunned with the massive impact of COVID-19, considering how quickly the virus propagated (Italy, Spain, France, the Netherlands), whereas other countries experienced a milder impact – all in all, this is a symmetric crisis that asks for joint reaction. If in an asymmetric crisis, such as the Eurozone crisis, the majority of the literature pledged for a comprehensive joint action at the level of EU institutions to address the crisis, there is enhanced ground for a response at the level of the EU when a symmetric crisis is at stake, at least from a theoretical point of view.

Since Chapter 1 only dwells on the theoretical considerations that underpin our methodology, we do not address the mismatch between desirability and feasibility. That is, we are only concerned with the delimitation of a theoretical framework that looks at objective conditions and lays down the foundation for solutions internally consistent with the objective conditions underlying the model. The problem is that, frequently, theory is not the perfect match with practice. In the EU, looking in retrospect, and going back to the theoretical underpinnings of European integration, that often happens. The purpose of the next chapters is to test our theoretical model against the imprints of reality on the multiple dimensions of the crisis that deserve careful analysis.

Chapter 2 encompasses a political and institutional analysis of the pandemic. At the beginning of the chapter, we address the political dimension of the severe public health crisis engendered by the pandemic. Public health policy ranks among the policies of the EU. It is nevertheless a timid policy area for the intervention of the EU, as the most important issues are still assigned to the national level. For this reason, it is important to take an overview on national governments' political reactions to the pandemic. Since it is not possible to analyse 27 member states, a sample of cases which we consider representative is selected. The obvious candidates are countries that were severely affected by COVID-19. The sudden development of the pandemic, after it was imported (so to speak) from China, is a fertile ground to understand how national authorities designed crisis management, and whether the answer prevented the virus from spreading at a tremendous speed.

At the same time, political decisions were taken at the level of the EU. What matters here is to understand if the EU level and the national level articulated in the face of the pandemic. The assessment of the EU is, however, constrained by the awareness of the limited role of the EU in this policy area. Evaluation must be restricted to the boundaries that constraint the EU action (supporting competences for the most part). Critically, we ask if EU institutions (notably those that are not controlled by member states) could have been more proactive crisis management agents. In theory, an obstacle surfaces when considering the hypothesis of a more proactive crisis manager EU: the early period of the pandemic brought with it an unprecedented scenario, one for which national authorities and EU institutions alike were not prepared to deal with. Some political inertia might be explained accordingly. At the same time, the crisis was perceived, right from the start, as a crisis that thwarted member states. Inward-looking governments neglected the condition of the pandemic as a transnational problem that touched all the member states. Absent awareness of the pandemic as a common problem is the ground for the lack of interaction (not to mention coordination, or even – as an ambitious hypothesis – harmonisation of efforts) between national governments, and their unwillingness to discuss joint action through the EU. The question that emerges is the following: was the political dimension of the crisis an obstacle to a comprehensive reaction to the pandemic?

Like it happened with the Eurozone crisis, institutional interaction, and in some cases the permeability of EU institutions to national interests, accounts an institutional dynamic where losers and winners come to the forefront. From the institutional point of view, this web of relationships brings to the surface implications for European integration per se. It all depends on the awareness of losers and winners, whether winners rank among institutions autonomous from the national authorities or the opposite. Pending on this assessment, conclusions must be drawn on a twofold dimension. First, the implications of the pandemic to the EU as a polity are under consideration: do we have more Europe or less Europe? Second, does the examination of losers and winners illustrate a new balance of powers within the institutional system of the EU? The combination of the aforementioned dimensions is also helpful: did the impact on the rebalancing of EU institutions produce an impact on European integration?

We assume that crises are the context for rising opportunities for institutional recalibration. Just as the Eurozone crisis produced a new balance of powers between the institutions of the EU (Vila Maior and Camisão, 2018), the question is whether institutional actors seized the opportunity to repositioning themselves. It is important to carefully observe institutional reactions to the events and to provide an interpretation of these movements. Sometimes, laggard, less influential institutions look at a crisis as an opportunity to gain influence in the chessboard. Thus, an important part of Chapter 2 pays attention to whether less influential institutions grabbed the opportunity to act proactively, anticipating future problems (perhaps, the European Commission and the EP). Conversely, it is important to judge interventions of institutions that are used to exert considerable influence in political and economic outcomes (the European Council and the ECB): were they as proactive as less influential institutions? If they were caught on the inertia trap, does that owe to their privileged position in the institutional system of the EU?

Chapter 3 unveils the economic dimension of the pandemic. This is a rich dimension of the crisis, although it was not the short-term priority when countries started to be affected by the spreading virus. As soon as a massive increase of spending was witnessed (due to contingency plans to address the implications of massive disease and of broad lockdown), and when governments' revenue was impacted because economic activity slowed down at once, macroeconomic consequences added to the crisis. The pandemic crisis is not only a public health emergency, but it also soon encompassed an economic dimension.

At the outset of the pandemic, governments and observers realised the likelihood of a twofold macroeconomic effect with a self-reinforcing dynamic. On the one hand, as economies plunged ruthlessly, revised macroeconomic forecasts pointed at a deep recession, with unemployment on the rise and a substantial drop of gross domestic product (GDP). Early estimations of the magnitude of the economic slowdown soon triggered the anxiety of economic policymakers at the national and the EU levels. On the other hand, fiscal policy effects were another reason of concern, especially because memories of the recent Eurozone crisis were still vivid. As a consequence of economic collapse and the ensuing recession, as well as of policy measures designed to prevent the virus from spreading (especially health-care spending), it became palpable that member states would be affected by fiscal policy unsustainability. This time, according to early estimations, fiscal policy indiscipline would hinder all member states at once, which reinforced the perception of the pandemic as a symmetric crisis.

Fiscal rules of the Eurozone were quickly suspended, so that national authorities were given leverage not only to address immediate challenges related with the financing of national healthcare systems but also to deal with the expected deterioration of the fiscal deficit. Nonetheless, threats were pending on some member states more than others for their public debt (un)sustainability. Highly indebted countries would face mounting pressures from financial markets, as public debt was expected to increase considerably. Again, the spectre of an asymmetric crisis resonates. In turn, this showcases how a symmetric crisis might turn into an asymmetric crisis if no appropriate measures are designed to prevent the crisis from undergoing this metamorphosis. Here, again, lessons from the recent Eurozone crisis come to the fore, as the likely implications of absent joint action at the EU level could be detrimental to some countries like they were in the recent Eurozone crisis.

The next three chapters encompass a sectoral dimension, as if they were case studies covering relevant topics of the pandemic. While the previous three chapters provided the macro framework for understanding the position of the EU in the context of the pandemic crisis, Chapters 4, 5, and 6 move to issue-focused aspects of the crisis. Nonetheless their specific, issue-oriented nature also impacted European integration. For this reason, they are relevant from the theoretical point of view since important consequences might be extracted for European integration.

In Chapter 4 we turn to a critical issue for crisis management: when national governments realised the severity of the pandemic, they decided, one after the other, to close borders. The underlying purpose was to isolate countries from the propagation of COVID-19. Movements of persons between member states were severely restricted. Differently, corridors were open to expedite the circulation of commodities across borders, thereby ensuring that one hallmark of European integration (the single market, notably the freedom of movement of commodities) was not jeopardised by the pandemic. From the perspective of a national government that aims at protecting the population from the outbreak of the virus, the measure seems understandable. The contagious potential of the virus was very high. One way to stop the virus from spreading from country to country was to impose border controls, with all the consequences attached (for instance, air traffic went to historical lows).

Yet, closing borders has an impact on the idiosyncrasy of European integration. Understandably, the two aspects interact at different levels. The freedom of movement of persons is a hallmark of European integration, something that is innate to the creation of the European Communities and was henceforth developed to ensure that not only workers but also persons as such enjoyed this freedom. Closing borders was an exceptional measure devised to stop the virus from spreading from country to country. We do not suggest that both aspects are in contradiction, as the rationale of border controls that prevent citizens from moving from one country to another is legitimate from the point of view of the rationale of crisis management. But we ask if the legitimate claim for security has once again paved the way to the much challenging path of securitisation. The aim of this chapter is to highlight a dimension that so far was absent from the analysis of European integration issues: the fragility of the EU – indeed, the fragility of nation-states – when affected by an exogenous crisis such as a pandemic.

It was expected that once the pandemic no longer affected Europe, national governments would abandon border controls and normality would be restored. Observers cannot escape the perception that exception might hurt fundamental values of European integration, such as the freedom of circulation of persons. As such, it is the EU, in a very important dimension of its ontology, that faces interruption while the pandemic lasts. One question of this chapter is whether the implementation of border controls represents a setback for European integration. The analysis moves on a fluid context, one that recognises the legitimacy of national governments to resort to border controls and to prevent non-nationals from coming into the country (and to prevent national citizens from going to foreign countries) but, at the same time, points at the incongruence of such measure when viewed from the perspective of the axiology of European integration.

Perhaps the analysis moves on a wrong template, as previous cases of border controls were exceptional, temporary and the underlying reasons legitimised by the legislation of the EU (for instance, according to legal provisions of the Schengen agreement, national governments might use border controls in specific circumstances). The EU was never faced by the prospect of a pandemic as with COVID-19. This is the rationale of exceptional measures that clash against the idiosyncrasy of European integration. Thus, the debate is between the awareness that exceptions are legitimate when critical values are at stake and the recognition that the EU is not a fragile polity when a basic value of European integration must undergo temporary interruption.

Chapter 5 deals with humanitarian emergency in the EU following the outbreak of the virus. The seriousness of the outbreak asked for contingency plans to mitigate the number of victims. Here again the initiative (and political leadership) was of national authorities. Different plans were designed, giving rise to an uncoordinated answer at the national level. At the first glance, each member state acted as if it was on its own. This also reflected the absence of political leadership of the EU. Since national governments decided that the appropriate answer to humanitarian emergency was national, they were hardly interested in submitting the issue to the Council of the EU (hereinafter Council). Other EU institutions, in turn, were limited not only by the initiative of national governments, but also because this is a policy area where the intervention of the EU is somewhat restricted.

The awareness of national solutions for the humanitarian emergency has implications for European integration as well. The sense of solidarity was largely absent. When Italy was troubled by the catastrophic consequences of a far-reaching outbreak of COVID-19, EU institutions neglected the request of assistance made by the Italian government. Only at a later stage, when Italy plunged into turmoil, the European Commission realised how wrong the absence was. At the same time, Germany accepted to receive some Italian patients in German hospitals, turning the page (but only timidly) on interstate solidarity during the pandemic crisis. Other member states also missed the plea for solidarity. They were anxious with the unprecedented effects of the pandemic. They therefore isolated from others, not only by closing borders but, crucially, by neglecting other countries' problems.

Paradoxically, a problem that affected all member states was not addressed through joint action. This conflicts with the established rationale of joint action, which is distinctive of European integration. Again, the exceptionality of the pandemic crisis was the original input for analysis, which disturbed the customary functioning of the EU. The discussion revolves around the consequences for European integration: was such inward, selfish position of national authorities consistent with the rationale of European integration? In addition, how did this stance impact on the external action of the EU (considering that internal disunion is not consistent with external union)? We take a cautious approach to the questions in Chapter 5. The key is the understanding that exceptional circumstances might legitimise exceptional measures, even those that apparently clash against the rationale of the EU. Whether this affects the embeddedness of the EU is a question that remains to be seen for the near future, when the ashes of turmoil settle down.

Amidst this spirit of national reassurance, the EU was not able to provide political leadership. Notwithstanding European Commission officials came frequently to the fore, this can hardly be understood as an evidence of political leadership of the EU. It sounded more a proof of life, which is understandable since the European Commission was appointed recently (four months before the outbreak of the pandemic in European territory) and political visibility and a sense of actorness was crucial in the first months on the institution. This nevertheless lags behind minimum requirements of political leadership. The chapter asks whether a correlation between national reassurance, absent solidarity at the EU level, and the lack of political leadership by the EU exists – an apparently unresolved tryptic stemming from the pandemic.

Chapter 6 addresses another exceptional circumstance owing to the reaction to the pandemic. Further constraints to the mobility of citizens were decided at the national level, when national governments realised the explosive contagious potential of the virus and, hence, forced citizens to lockdown. For that purpose, national governments resorted to the state of exception, giving rise to the temporary denial of basic fundamental rights. According to national governments, the state of constitutional exceptionalism was justified on grounds of the urgency to contain the propagation of the virus. Constitutional exceptionalism is a breach on constitutional guarantees afforded to citizens, but this is hardly envisaged as a breach on the constitution itself (at least for authors who legitimised the declaration of the state of emergency).

A deeper review is necessary, though. There was no consensus on the declaration of constitutional exceptionalism as the appropriate measure to contain the virus by forcing citizens' reclusion. Critics claim that proportionality was not respected and that the state of emergency was premature and not reasoned. Future unintended effects of the state of exception with constitutional backup are at stake. Critics acknowledge that formal mechanisms act as a guarantee against the abuses of constitutional exceptionalism. Parliaments have the final say on the approval of the state of exception. The institution that closely represents citizens decides whether citizens must endure limited, or even restricted, fundamental rights for the sake of a superior goal. Maybe this is not enough, especially when governments increasingly resort to exceptions to temporarily derogate fundamental values.

The issue bears importance for European integration. One fundamental value of European integration is the rule of law and established fundamental rights assigned to citizens by the EU's constitutional settlement. It must be remembered that the EU turned into a legal provision of its own the respect of the rule of law and fundamental individual rights when examining whether applicant countries were eligible to EU membership. As in the previous two chapters, decisions approved at the national level have an impact on European integration. Needless to say, EU institutions have no responsibility, nor do they have a say, when a country ponders the possibility of enforcing constitutional exceptionalism. Yet, since the EU is not disconnected from member states, and indeed member states still play an influential role in the configuration of EU policies, the question is whether the state of constitutional exceptionalism also hampers the EU.

The research hypothesis is whether the contamination of the EU by constitutional exceptionalism should be disregarded because of the broader sense of exceptionalism triggered by the pandemic. Non-conventional approaches of law are added to the analysis. They move within a different analytical framework. The awareness that non-conventional sources of justice come to the forefront, and their connection to a volatile nature of the law in response to changing social circumstances, brings a new scenario to the analysis. This innovative analytical framework must be compared with the conventional model of constitutionalism and to the strict obeyance to the rule of law, and whether, for both approaches, constitutional exceptionalism is acceptable as a demanding precondition for the adjustment of law to temporary anomalies in the society. The EU cannot escape this discussion, not only for the embeddedness on the rule of law, but also because the EU has its own legal system with many formal similarities with member states' legal systems. Danger comes from the perception that even the EU might accept constitutional exceptionalism and whether this clashes against member states' political willingness at a certain moment.

In the concluding chapter, we summarise the main findings. After briefly reviewing the conclusion of each chapter, we provide a broad assessment that aims at answering our main research question: did the EU perform well as a crisis manager in the initial stages of the pandemic crisis? Since this is a broad, evaluative question, five subsidiary research questions will also be taken into consideration:

(i) Was economic policy consistent with the challenges stemming from the crisis?
(ii) Did the pandemic trigger an institutional recalibration of the EU institutional system?
(iii) Was it possible to overcome national unilateralism and bring the EU to the centre of the stage?
(iv) Did exceptionalism (border controls, humanitarian emergency feeding national reassurance and constitutionalism exceptionalism) hinder

European integration? If so, are negative implications bound to be transitory?

(v) In the current state of the pandemic, do we have more Europe or less Europe?

Notes

1 According to the International Monetary Fund, "[i]t is very likely that this year the global economy will experience its worst recession since the Great Depression (…)". IMF 2020. World Economic Outlook Chapter 1 The Great Lockdown, April 2020, p. v. Available online at www.imf.org/en/Publications/WEO/Issues/2020/04/14/weo-april-2020 [Accessed 16 April 2020].

2 Critical juncture is a core concept of historical institutionalism that refers to brief and exceptional phases of institutional flux during which more significant change is possible (Capoccia and Kelemen, 2007).

3 Euobserver. "Merkel: Virus is biggest challenge in EU history", 7 April 2020. Available online at https://euobserver.com/coronavirus/148003 [Accessed 8 April 2020].

Bibliography

Boin, A., Ekengren, M., and Rhinard, M., 2020. Hiding in Plain Sight: Conceptualizing the Creeping Crisis. *Risks, Hazards & Crisis in Public Policy*, 11(2), pp. 116–38.

Capoccia, G. and Kelemen, D., 2007. The Study of Critical Junctures: Theory, Narrative and Counterfactuals in Historical Institutionalism. *World Politics*, 59(3), pp. 341–69.

Milward, A., 1999. *The European Rescue of the Nation State*. London: Routledge.

Nanopoulos, E. and Vergis, F., 2019. Introduction: The Elephant in the Room: A Tale of Crisis. In E. Nanopoulos and F. Vergis, eds. *The Crisis behind the Eurocrisis: The Eurocrisis as a Multidimensional Systemic Crisis of the EU*. Cambridge: Cambridge University Press, pp. 1–22.

Streeck, W. and Thelen, K., 2005. Introduction: institutional change in advanced political economies. In W. Streeck and K. Thelen, eds. *Beyond Continuity: Institutional Change in Advanced Political Economies*. Oxford: Oxford University Press, pp. 3–39.

Vila Maior, P. and Camisão, I., 2018. Eurozone Governance in the Aftermath of the Crisis: A Proxy for a New Institutional Balance? In J. M. Caetano and M. R. Sousa, ed. *Challenges and Opportunities for Eurozone Governance*, New York: Nova Science, pp. 97–119.

1 A crisis beyond the crisis

1.1 Introduction

The process of European integration has been marked by many crises. However, the ongoing pandemic crisis has some particularities that set it apart from previous crises. This singularity, we argue, could have an impact on the processes of response to the crisis and policy change. Chapter 1 unveils the theoretical framework of the book. Section 1.2 builds on the burgeoning literature on crisis to reflect on the relation between crisis and reform and introduces the theoretical rationale for assessing change, based on an adaptation of the model proposed by Streeck and Thelen (2005). Section 1.3 draws a comparison between two previous crises (Eurozone and migration crises) and the pandemic crisis. Section 1.4 shows that a key dissimilarity is the symmetry of the pandemic crisis, as opposed to the asymmetric nature of the previous ones. The main argument of the chapter hence rests on the idea that this symmetry enhances the ground for a response at the level of the EU, at least from a theoretical point of view. Since Chapter 1 only dwells on the theoretical considerations that underpin our methodology, the purpose of the next chapters of the book is to test the theoretical framework we propose here against the imprints of reality on the multiple dimensions of the crisis that deserve careful analysis.

1.2 Crisis and reform: paths of continuity and discontinuity

Crisis is part of the EU lexicon almost from the beginning and, in fact, the idea that crises could act as a propelling force to the process of European integration, embodied in the well-known line attributed to Jean Monnet (1978),[1] is largely accepted as evidence in the EU literature. Arguably, Monnet's sentence is aligned with the historical institutionalist approach that maintains that a crisis could represent a 'critical juncture'[2] (Collier and Collier, 1991; 2002; Capoccia and Kelemen, 2007; Capoccia, 2015), that is, an exceptional (and brief) phase of institutional flux during which more significant change is possible (Capoccia and Kelemen, 2007, p. 341). Even though generally historical institutionalists devote most of their attention to continuity and

DOI: 10.4324/9781003153900-2

equilibrium, rather than to change, some works, notably macrohistorical analyses that focus on the development of polities, acknowledge the fact that institutional trajectories could deviate during critical junctures (Capoccia and Kelemen, 2007, p. 342). Critical junctures are therefore

> moments in which uncertainty as to the future of an institutional arrangement allows for political agency and choice to play a decisive causal role in setting an institution on a certain path of development, a path that then persists over a long period of time.
>
> (Capoccia, 2015, pp. 2–3)

Indeed, by representing a phase of disorder in the normal functioning of a system – one that entails the perception of a threat to the fundamental values and basic structures of a system, profound uncertainty and a sense of urgency in the response (Boin et al., 2005; Boin, 't Hart and Kuipers, 2017) – a crisis frequently exposes the insufficiencies of the system, not only to deal with unexpected challenges, but also to operate at the best of its capabilities. In a nutshell, a crisis could lead to a transformation in an otherwise stable and resistant to change institutional and policy path. Confirming this line of reasoning, the literature on policy reform and organisational change has shown that crises generate a window of opportunity for reforming institutional structures and long-standing policies (Kingdon, 2003; Cortell and Peterson, 1999). Arguably, the so-called crisis-reform thesis (Boin and 't Hart, 2000) adds a positive dimension to an obvious negative and disruptive one, as it considers that, by triggering a process of deinstitutionalisation, crises may open the door to a long-needed institutional renewal, which would be extremely difficult in normal times:

> [t]he way policy decisions are made, the ranking of policy goals, the daily routines and patterns of authority – all these institutionalised features of public administration and the policy process became subject to discussion.
>
> (Boin and 't Hart, 2000, p. 12)

However, the degree and nature of this transformation might vary significantly, ranging from 'restoring order' (a conservative approach) to revitalisation and institutional redesign (a reformist approach). Whereas the later aims to rebalance or to redesign the institutional features of the policy sector in order to adapt them to the new environment, the former aims to maintain the institutional essence (Boin and 't Hart, 2000, p. 21). Although in theory both conservative and reformist approaches have fairly similar chances of succeeding or failing, the literature on crisis management has highlighted that overcoming the many existing barriers to institutional change in policymaking is far from being an easy task (Boin and 't Hart, 2000; 2003). This might explain why so often crisis leaders choose to defend (rather than to reform) the existing institutions and policies. It might also shed light on a fairly conservative structure of polities and of the political process: even faced with a critical juncture, where the window of opportunity to change is open, institutions and policies are not changed.

At this point, it is worth noting that although a crisis could unfold a substantial reform of the system that is disrupted by it, this reform does not necessarily occur. Trying to make sense of very different outcomes, when it comes to change, emerging from events that have been classified as crisis, Boin, 't Hart and McConnel (2009) advanced a possible explanation based on a crisis exploitation model.[3] For them, actors who seek to exploit the crisis-induced opportunity space (to strengthen their positions, to attract or deflect public attention, to reform old policies or to create new ones) get involved in frame contests concerning the nature and severity of the crisis, who is to blame and the right path to the future. The goal is to have their frame accepted as the dominant 'crisis narrative', which in turn could help to push for non-incremental changes in policy fields otherwise very resistant to change (Boin, 't Hart and McConnell, 2009, p. 4).

On the topic of institutional change, and more specifically on the question of the type of change that might occur, Streeck and Thelen (2005) warned for the limits of models of change that compartmentalise institutional stability and institutional change and ignore the capacity of endogenous factors for triggering a significant transformation. Far-reaching change is not always the result of abrupt and exogenous factors, but can also be the result of the accumulation of small, frequently seemingly insignificant adjustments (Streeck and Thelen, 2005, p. 8). The authors propose an operative model that distinguishes between processes of change, which can be incremental or abrupt, and results of change, which might amount to either continuity or discontinuity (see Table 1.1). The main argument is that historical breakpoints do not necessarily lead to discontinuity, as often there is an urge to survive and return (to the status quo) and that in fact transformative change (in the model referred as 'gradual transformation', which is also a type of discontinuity) could result from incremental, creeping change (Streeck and Thelen, 2005). Arguably, the first claim is in line with the conservative approach, which asserts that more frequently than probably expected (considering the mainstream crisis-reform

Table 1.1 Streeck and Thelen (2005) model of change

		Results of change	
		Continuity	*Discontinuity*
Processes of change	Incremental	Reproduction by adaptation	Gradual transformation
	Abrupt	Survival and return	Breakdown and replacement

Source: Reproduced from Streeck and Thelen (2005, p. 9).

thesis) leaders are more eager to return to the 'certainty' of the pre-crisis situation than to take a leap of faith to the 'uncertainty' of a radically new policy or institutional design.

Turning now our attention to the EU's specific case, a quick overview of the history of European integration shows that several crises (that occurred inside and outside EU's borders) have triggered important opportunities for developments in the institutional architecture, in the decision-making procedures and in the expansion of the overall areas of competence of the EU. However, as regards the results of change, although frequently the proposals point to the 'breakdown and replacement' result, the actual outcome is more in line with the 'gradual transformation' hypothesis. Put it differently, although generally crisis have clearly signalled the need for a (deep) reform of the EU policies and procedures, not every crisis has led to a significant or rapid deepening of the European project. Actually, some crises even marked a setback or at least a stalemate in the integration process, as was the case of the so-called empty chair crisis (1965) or the Constitutional Treaty crisis (2005).

That being said, some EU supranational institutions, particularly the European Commission (henceforth Commission), have been keen in grasping the opportunity opened by crisis events to push forward the integration process, issuing proposals that often aim for a 'break and replacement' type of change. Even though this 'purposeful opportunism' (Cram, 1994) and 'policy entrepreneurship' (Kingdon, 2003) might not be sufficient to secure a radical transformation of the policy area, it normally accelerates the pace of incremental change, preventing 'a survival and return' result. What is more, if it is true that European integration has evolved mostly through incremental change, it seems also fair to assume that crisis, rather than a grain of sand in the gear, represents the oil that maintains the wheel in motion. In this sense, building on Streeck and Thelen's model as regards abrupt processes of change, but adapting it to the subject of this book, we add another layer to the axis of results, which tentatively we name *push forward*. Our argument is that although crises in the EU may not necessarily lead to abrupt change, they generally boost incremental change, therefore accelerating EU's transformation. Additionally, and considering the complexity of the EU decision-making process, we believe it is useful to distinguish between the type of change envisioned by the proposals initially made to respond to the crisis (which frequently aim for a 'breakdown and replacement' type of result) and the type of change that resulted from the decision actually taken (that tends to be more conservative and incremental) (see Table 1.2).

Yet, adding to the complexity of the analysis, at least since 2008 the EU has been experiencing an abnormal number of crises, which means that the combined results of these multiple crises could trigger significant changes on how the EU functions, in what Rhinard (2019, p. 617) has labelled 'crisification' of EU policymaking. For the author, a sort of crisis-oriented mode has an impact not only on the nature of the processes by which collective decisions

Table 1.2 Adaptation from Streeck and Thelen (2005) model of change

		Type of Change					
		Proposal			*Decision*		
		Continuity	*Discontinuity*		*Continuity*	*Discontinuity*	
Processes of change	Abrupt	Survival and return	Breakdown and replacement	Push forward (boost incremental change)	Survival and return	Breakdown and replacement	Push forward (boost incremental change)

Source: Authors.

are made, but also on our understanding of those processes. Thus, as a result of this sequency of crises, the EU policymaking is today characterised by

> a determined focus on finding the next urgent event, a prioritization of speed in decision-making, new perceptions of which actors matter, and new narratives on the role and purpose of the EU.
>
> (Rhinard, 2019, p. 629)

Indeed, in the last decade – suggestively referred as the 'age of crises' (Dinan, Nugent and Paterson, 2016, p. 1) – a significant number of disruptive events exerted continuous pressure over EU's leadership. The EU's response capacity was pushed to its limits by an increasing number of internal crises, including the economic and financial crisis, and the subsequent sovereign debt and Eurozone crises, the migration crisis, the (endless) Brexit negotiations, repeated terrorists attacks, violations of the rule of law in some member states or the rise of divisive nationalism; but also of external tests, namely the uncertainty of the transatlantic partnership due to the 'erratic' foreign policy of the Trump administration, the rise of China, the confrontational external policy of Russia and the invasion of parts of the Ukrainian territory, the instability in EU's neighbourhood and the stalemate of the enlargement policy adding to the instability of Southern Balkans.

These massive challenges lead some authors to consider that for quite some time now the EU is operating in a context of permanent crisis or 'perennial crisis' (Nanopoulos and Vergis, 2019), and therefore it is also in a 'permanent crisis' management mode, which supports Rhinard's argument. Dinan, Nugent and Paterson (2016, pp. 4–5) identified three general sources of the EU's state of crisis: the weak foundations of some aspects of the EU's system of governance (including the absence of clear, accountable leadership) and of some core EU policies (such as the Economic and Monetary Union and the Schengen agreement), the significant differences between member states as regards national needs and preferences, and the sensibility of the EU to what happens in the international system, that is, the sensibility to external factors.

Whereas this 'polycrisis' (Zeitlin, Nicoli and Laffan, 2019) environment is not necessarily enough to fundamentally reshape the direction of European integration, it certainly contributes to alter the pace of European integration in several policy areas. In this book we will zoom in the multiple layers of the ongoing pandemic crisis. Throughout the next chapters we will use our adaption of the Streeck and Thelen's model to assess change (or the proposal of it) resulting from this still unfolding crisis. Before doing so, we believe it is important to explore the particular nature of the pandemic crisis, which, we argue, is different from previous crises. A key dissimilarity is the initial symmetry of the pandemic crisis, as opposed to the mostly asymmetric nature of the previous ones.

The main argument of the chapter rests on the idea that symmetry enhances the ground for a response at the level of the EU, at least from a theoretical point of view. To prove our argument, in Section 1.3 we will draw a brief comparison between two major previous crises – the Eurozone crisis and the migration crisis – and the pandemic crisis. Since the purpose of the book is to analyse the pandemic crisis, we will draw on the burgeoning literature on the Eurozone and the migration crises to trace their profile.

1.3 What does this crisis have in common with previous ones? A comparison with the Eurozone and the migration crises

Like the ongoing pandemic, the Eurozone crisis was a multidimensional, 'mutating' crisis that operated on different levels (global, EU, member states) and different dimensions (banking and financial, economic, sovereign debt) (Dyson, 2016, p. 55). The origins of the crisis can be traced back to the accelerated decline of housing and subprime mortgages markets in the United States and, more specifically, to the collapse of the Lehman Brothers in September 2008, the fourth-largest US investment bank. The immediate result was the global economic downturn. The waves of shock hit the EU in 2009–2010, testing the foundations of one of the most recognised and praised achievements of the European construction, the Economic and Monetary Union (EMU). EMU bluntly failed the test. Built on the premise that it would facilitate economic convergence among participating countries and accelerated economic growth, and hence a more homogenous economic area, EMU had arguably the opposite result with the economies of Eurozone countries further diverging and experience at best modest growth (Dinan, Nugent and Paterson, 2016, p. 2).

However, precisely because member states had fundamental differences as regards the strength of national economies and the state of national finances, the Eurozone crisis was from the start 'a phenomenon of attribution' (Dyson, 2016, p. 56), meaning that the answer to the question of who was to blame was greatly disputed, ranging from exogenous factors (rooted in the US crisis), to individual reckless financial behaviour of some member states, to the eventual recognition of design failures of EMU. Although closely associated to a global financial crisis and having led to a generalised recession in the Eurozone and in fact in the EU as a whole, the Eurozone crisis started as a sovereign debt crisis in one member state of EMU – Greece – that spilled over to the Greek banking system (Gibson, Palivos and Tavlas, 2013). Eventually, the crisis extended to other Eurozone countries such as Ireland, Portugal, Cyprus, Spain and Italy and became known as the Eurozone crisis, which was a combination of government debt and banking crises (Tosun, Wetzel and Zapryanova, 2014).

Although the sovereign debt crisis and the weakness of banking systems were from the start acknowledged as a serious risk to the whole Eurozone (European Central Bank, 2010) and indeed the recession affected the whole area, the Eurozone crisis, despite it all-encompassing name, was never perceived as a truly symmetric crisis, as the negative spillover effects of significant structural rigidities and imbalances between Eurozone member states (Cox, 2015) eventually transformed the crisis into a crisis of the Southern countries. Indeed, the idea that member states most affected by the crisis were to blame for their own situation became the dominant narrative for a considerable period of time, leading to a sort of 'naming and shaming' attitude that was received with extreme dissatisfaction in the countries mostly affected by the devastating effects of crisis.

The Eurozone crisis thus potentiated pre-existent divisions in Europe between creditor and debtor member states, rich and poor, North and South. The recipe for exiting the crisis, based on severe austerity measures that aggravated the social dimension of the crisis to the point of clearly hampering citizens' fundamental rights (European Parliament, 2015), further escalated divisions. As Cox (2015, p. 12) noted, eventually it fuelled a sort of 'lose-lose discourse of victimhood' with citizens of the creditor member states perceiving themselves as victims of the Southern rule-breaking, obliged to pay a bill they did not sign for, and citizens of the debtor member states perceiving themselves as exhausted by endless and ruthless austerity measures, obliged to pay a bill that ought to be endorsed to the banking system. As a result, social unrest across the EU became frequent, public trust in national and EU institutions decreased and the support for extremist parties was boosted (Tosun, Wetzel and Zapryanova, 2014).

Like the Eurozone crisis, the migration crisis (also known as the refugee crisis) had external triggers, namely the growing instability in Europe's neighbourhood, while putting to the test (and eventually disclosing the fragility of) several internal areas, such as free movement of people, the Schengen agreement or internal security. As with the Eurozone crisis, it also brought to the daylight profound differences between member states in terms of preferences and goals, fuelling a 'East–West split' (Monar, 2016, pp. 137–8) and casting doubts regarding the humanitarian dimension of the European project, as well as regarding the basilar principle of solidarity between member states.

Although migration is not necessarily a problem, and in fact could be a solution particularly considering that many developed countries (European countries included) are experiencing a steady decline in birth rates and the consequent ageing of their population,[4] over the last decades the scale and scope of migration has changed, and the number of forcibly displaced persons has grown substantially. From the 1990s onwards, the flow of persons seeking EU's protection increased considerably, first as a result of the disintegration of the former Soviet Union and of Yugoslavia and afterwards due to war-torn in countries such as Syria, Afghanistan and Iraq.

The former Third Pillar of Maastricht – Justice and Home Affairs – gradually evolved from intergovernmental to supranational decision-making, but the attempts to build a common approach to visas, immigration and asylum have somewhat fallen short (Staab, 2011, p. 143), partly because some member states were more concerned to 'dodge the bullet' than to find a cohesive (joint) solution to the problem. The exceptions granted to some member states and concerns over sovereignty resulted in the coexistence of different standards across the EU.

The shortcomings of the EU migration policy and particularly of the Common European Asylum System (CEAS) became clear in more recent years, when an upsurge of migrants fled to Europe by crossing the Mediterranean. Many of them were reported missing or dead. Although previous dramatic events (namely in 2013) had put migration under the spotlights, the year of 2015 is generally identified as a turning point as an unusual number of migrants, the majority of which asylum-seekers fleeing for war in Syria, Iraq and other countries, arrived in the EU. In face of this unprecedented wave, the limits of the legal procedures in place to respond to asylum-seekers, namely the Dublin Regulation III (that came into force in 2013), rapidly became undeniable. Although the Regulation lists a set of criteria to identify the EU country responsible for examining an asylum application (such as family unity, possession of residence documents or visas, irregular entry or stay and visa-waived entry), in practice the criterion more often used is irregular entry, meaning that the member state through which the asylum-seeker first entered the EU become responsible for examining the claim (Radjenovic, 2019). Considering that in 2015 and 2016 almost one million people (asylum-seekers and other migrants) arrived in the EU (European Commission, 2017), the generalised use of this criterion added unbearable pressure on some member states (especially Greece, but also Italy, Spain and Malta) that are natural states of arrival for geographical reasons.

The immediate reaction of neighbouring states was to close borders. Thus, as Dinan, Nugent and Paterson (2016, p. 1) noted, one visible consequence of the migration crisis was the severe limitation on free movement within the EU and, consequently, a partial breakdown of the Schengen agreement. Additionally, different narratives regarding the crisis emerged, unveiling deep divergences between member states as regards the issue of migration and the best solution to tackle the crisis. Those differences eventually blocked important pieces of the comprehensive reform of the migration policy proposed by the Juncker Commission. Whereas some member states (such as Germany) and some EU institutions (namely the Commission and the EP), emphasised the need to reform the procedures to enable a common *European* response, others, headed by the so-called Visegrad Group (Poland, Hungary, Czech Republic and Slovakia), denied the existence of a European crisis and emphasised *national* measures, including the criminalisation of irregular migrants. Ultimately, this clash resulted in "an increased externalisation of the European migration and asylum policy (…) to partly compensate for the failure of the internal measures." (Schramm, 2019, pp. 10–11), of which the EU–Turkey agreement[5] was an example.

The ensuing pandemic crisis shares with the two crises described above some features. First, it had an external trigger. It began as a health disease,[6] a new coronavirus, that originated outside Europe. Despite some contradictory information regarding the origin of the virus, the original source of the outbreak is traced back to December 2019 in Wuhan, in China (World Health Organization, 2020, p. 1). Secondly, it developed into an overarching multidimensional crisis with potential destructive effects that extend well beyond the original problem – public health safety – pervading social, political, economic, legal and institutional arenas. Thirdly, notwithstanding its rapid spreading, it only fully captured the attention of the European leaders when the disease had already crossed European borders. According to Boin, Ekengren and Rhinard (2020), the current pandemic is yet another example of the complex problems (hard to define and hard to manage) that characterise modern society. Building on the differences between two ideal types of crises – 'fast-burning crisis' (with a clear beginning and end) and 'slow-burning crisis' (with no clear beginning or end) – the authors suggest the concept of 'creeping crisis' to describe many of the contemporary problems:

> a threat to widely shared societal values or life-sustaining systems that evolves over time and space, is foreshadowed by precursor events, subject to varying degrees of political and/or societal attention, and impartially or insufficiently addressed by authorities.
>
> (Boin, Ekengren and Rhinard, 2020, p. 122)

Creeping crises have therefore both a temporal and a spatial dimension. From the temporal perspective, since they may incubate during long periods of time, with unclear beginnings and ends, suddenly manifesting themselves, they could be classified as slow-burning crisis with incidental 'sparking'. From a spatial perspective, they often originated in distant locations as a result of transboundary processes or apparently unrelated policy domains, before they 'explode' into a regional or local crisis. For the authors, these crises should not be regarded as exceptional events clearly limited in time or space, but instead 'as permanent global threats that can manifest themselves as seemingly acute crises at the local level' (Boin, Ekengren and Rhinard, 2020, p. 120); in sum, they are crises that arrive slowly and are slow to leave (Boin, Lodge and Luesink, 2020).

To fit this categorisation, the current pandemic crisis must be understood within a broader framework that entails complex societal threats, such as public health threats, resulting from accelerated globalisation. Considered as a sign of civilisational progress, globalisation has positively impacted on people's lives, for example by reducing the costs of moving people, goods, money and information (Fugita and Hamaguchi, 2020) and therefore facilitating (and democratising) access to different products and services. However, on the flipside, globalisation potentiated local, regional and international inequalities (or at least highlighted the existent ones), leading to high concentration of population in urban areas, a greater concentration of economic activities in specific regions and increased fluxes of international economic migration. Moreover, boosted mobility that resulted from the reduction of transportation costs (with the positive impact of opening and 'shrinking' the world) also facilitated the rapid spread of viruses, of which the ongoing pandemic crisis is just an example (Fugita and Hamaguchi, 2020). Due to its global impact, the COVID-19 pandemic amplified the visibility of this paradox, fuelling (old) debates on alternative scenarios for the post-crisis world:

> The pandemic is exposing weaknesses, as well as strengths, within our societies, government structures and systems, calling for critical reflection to map our way forward.
>
> (Oosterhof, 2020)

1.4 What sets the pandemic apart? Symmetry and cooperation

It is precisely its truly global spreading that sets the current pandemic crisis aside from previous ones. Unlike other crises, even crisis that were named 'global' (such as the global financial crisis), the COVID-19 pandemic really affected all countries with very few exceptions,[7] and more than 127 million people around the world,[8] being a perfect example of a 'problem without passport'[9], that is, a challenge that disregards national borders threatening people in many different nation-states (Johnson, 2020, p. E148). Also, as Fugita and Hamaguchi (2020) noted, contrary to other infectious diseases, this pandemic has not a direct connection to poor environments. It is therefore a 'global symmetric crisis' (European Commission, 2020), not only as the health issue concerns, but also as regards the economic shock that resulted from the initial public health crisis (Botta, Caverzasi and Russo, 2020; Celi, Guarascio and Somonazzi, 2020; Eurogroup, 2020; Herrero, 2020) that cut across countries with very different social, economic and political characteristics, even if its short- to medium-term consequences might be profoundly asymmetric, unveiling how fragile and unprepared some countries are to handle the multidimensional effects of the crisis.

Considering that the unevenness of previous crises (such as the Eurozone or the migration crises) have served to stiffen differences between member states, pointing to disaggregation (Dinan, Nugent and Paterson, 2016, p. 9), we are interested in examining if and how the current crisis has helped to overcome the frequent clash between wealthier and poorer EU member states (or in its oversimplified version, net contributors versus net recipients), hence favouring cooperative solutions. For the purpose of this analysis, we use the concept of cooperation advanced by Keohane (1984, p. 51):

> [c]ooperation occurs when actors adjust their behavior to the actual or anticipated preferences of the others, through a process of policy coordination.

Although Keohane was referring to the frequently self-interested process that pushes states to create international regimes, we find this definition broad enough to encompass both 'egoistic cooperation' (the one moved by rational self-interested states) as well as cooperation moved from common bonds and the idea of a common good. Building on the bourgeoning literature on global problems – that is, problems that affect the interests of many states, peoples and nations (Roder, 1985, pp. 35–6) – that generally claims that this kind of problems require international cooperation (Roder, 1985), our argument is that the uncommon symmetry of the current pandemic should foster cooperation among EU member states, thereby enabling common responses, through policy coordination, and possibly unblocking change.

It is true that the literature on collective action and international cooperation also points to the difficulties associated to cooperation between a large number of states (Keohane, 1984; Axelrod and Keohane, 1985; Axelrod, 2000). In this regard, it could be argued that membership of the EU should, on its own, foster cooperation, as several characteristics identified in the literature as facilitating cooperation, even in the confrontational context of international anarchy (Axelrod, 1984; Axelrod and Keohane, 1985) are present, including the fact that interactions between member states take place within a strong (and in this case actually constraining, considering the level of power delegation in EU institutions) institutional context, which in turn might lengthen what Axelrod named 'the shadow of the future'[10] and the idea of reciprocity. Despite the favourable environment, cooperation within the EU is far from being exempt of hurdles. And yet, arguably a symmetric crisis could help overcoming a fundamental hurdle to cooperation, in Axelrod's (2000) words 'the problem of cooperation', that is, the tension between what is good for the individual actor in the short run and what is good for the group in the long run. What is more, if states are experiencing the same crisis at the same time, arguably they perceive the payoffs of their decision as being also symmetrical. Using the prisoner's dilemma as model, some studies show that 'symmetry has a positive effect on mutual cooperation whereas asymmetry substantially decreases cooperation rates' (Beckenkamp, Hennig-Schmidt and Maier-Rigaud, 2006, p. 3).

Even though initially the responses to the public health crisis were disarticulated, national (not to mention local) solutions and unilateral remedies, rapidly mechanisms of European integration were brought to the fore and established patters of governance in the EU drew attention to solutions at the supranational level. Managing the COVID-19 crisis has turned up to be a colossal test to national governments. When faced with a crisis, policymakers have four challenging crucial tasks: sense-making (understanding a crisis); making critical decisions and solving the immediate problems; communicate effectively; devising 'exit strategies' to end the crisis (Boin, Lodge and Luesink, 2020, p. 190). However,

> [t]he 'creeping' characteristics of the pandemic posed novel and complex challenges, even to those policy-makers well-versed in the management of 'acute' crises, such as plane crashes or natural disasters.
>
> (Boin, Lodge and Luesink, 2020, p. 190)

Besides the shortage of information about the nature of the virus, which amplified the difficulty to craft adequate responses, the length of the crisis led to a sort of extended 'crisis regime' (Boin, Lodge and Luesink, 2020) that is testing the resilience of both national political leaders and citizens. In this scenario, European (and international) cooperation gained renewed relevance. Also, the perceived symmetry of the crisis should have blocked the use of a sort of 'naming and shaming' strategy that was common in other crises (such as the two abovementioned) and that eventually increased the divisions between member states, preventing or delaying important reforms. In the following chapters, we will test our theoretical argument against the supranational and national responses to the crisis, assessing patterns of continuity or discontinuity stemming from the ongoing pandemic.

Notes

1 'Europe will be forged in crises, and will be the sum of the solutions adopted for those crises' (Monnet, 1978, p. 417).
2 Actually, the literature uses the concepts of 'turning point', 'crisis' or 'unsettled times' as synonyms of 'critical junctures' (Capoccia and Kelemen, 2007, p. 341).
3 The authors define crisis' exploitation as 'the purposeful utilisation of crisis-type rhetoric to significantly alter levels of political support for incumbent public office-holders and existing public policies and their alternatives' (Boin, 't Hart and McConnell, 2009, p. 5).
4 The 2030 Agenda for sustainable development recognises the contribution of migration to sustainable development and the importance of planned and well-managed migration policies. See www.un.org/en/sections/issues-depth/migration/index.html
5 The EU-Turkey Statement.
6 SARS-CoV-2.
7 See WHO Coronavirus Disease (COVID-19) Dashboard. Available at: https://covid19.who.int [Accessed 1 November 2020].
8 See ECDC. COVID-19 Situation Update Worldwide, As of Week 12, Updated 1 April 2021. Available at: www.ecdc.europa.eu/en/geographical-distribution-2019-ncov-cases [Accessed 8 April 2021].
9 The expression was coined by the former United Nations Secretary, Kofi Annan (2009) to refer to problems such as pollution, organised crime, or the proliferation of deadly weapons that require collective action, though multilateral fora such as international organisations.
10 According to Axelrod (1984), the shadow of the future must be sufficiently large for cooperation, that is, 'the importance of the next encounter between the same two individuals must be great enough to make defection an unprofitable strategy' (Axelrod, 1984, p. 4).

Bibliography

Axelrod, R., 1984. *The Evolution of Cooperation*, New York: Basic Books.
Axelrod, K., 2000. On Six Advances in Cooperation Theory. *Analyse & Kritik*, 22, pp. 130–1, Available at: www-personal.umich.edu/~axe/research/SixAdvances.pdf. [Accessed 28 November 2020].

Axelrod, R. and Keohane, R. O., 1985. Achieving Cooperation under Anarchy: Strategies and Institutions. *World Politics*, 38(1), pp. 226–54.

Beckenkamp, M., Hennig-Schmidt, H. and Maier-Rigaud, F., 2006. Cooperation in symmetric and asymmetric prisoner's dilemma games. *Max-Planck-Institute for Research on Collective Goods*, Working Paper No. 2006–25.

Boin, A., Ekengren, M., and Rhinard, M., 2020. Hiding in Plain Sight: Conceptualizing the Creeping Crisis. *Risks, Hazards & Crisis in Public Policy*, 11(2), pp. 116–38.

Boin, A., Lodge, M. and Luesink, M., 2020. Learning from the COVID-19 Crisis: An Initial Analysis of National Responses. *Policy Design and Practice*, 3(3), pp. 189–204, DOI: https://doi.org/10.1080/25741292.2020.1823670.

Boin, A. and 't Hart, P., 2000. Institutional Crisis and Reforms in Policy Sectors. In: H. Wagenaar, ed. *Government Institutions: Effects, Changes and Normative Foundations*. New York: Springer, pp. 9–31.

Boin, A., 't Hart, P. and Kuipers, S., 2017. The Crisis Approach. In: H. Rodríguez, H. Quarantelli and R. R. Dynes, eds. *Handbook of Disaster Research*. New York, Springer, pp. 23–38.

Boin, A., 't Hart, P. and McConnell, A., 2009. Crisis Exploitation: Political and Policy Impacts of Framing Contests. *Journal of European Public Policy*, 16(1), pp. 81–106.

Boin, A., 't Hart, P., Stern, E. and Sundelius, B., 2005. *The Politics of Crisis Management: Public Leadership Under Stress*. Cambridge: Cambridge University Press.

Botta, A., Caverzasi, E. and Russo, A., 2020. Fighting the COVID-19 Crisis: Debt Monetisation and EU Recovery Bonds. *Review of European Economic Policy*, 55(4), pp. 239–244. Available at: www.intereconomics.eu/pdf-download/year/2020/number/4/article/fighting-the-covid-19-crisis-debt-monetisation-and-eu-recovery-bonds.html. [Accessed 27 November 2020].

Capoccia, G., 2015. Critical Junctures and Institutional Change. Paper prepared for inclusion in: J. Mahoney, and K. Thelen, eds. *Advances in Comparative Historical Analysis in the Social Sciences*. Cambridge: Cambridge University Press. Available at: https://pdfs.semanticscholar.org/fa79/fde0ca78361bdcd89a1ad3606c2a8e3af45e.pdf. [Accessed 12 December 2020].

Capoccia, G. and Kelemen, D., 2007. The Study of Critical Junctures: Theory, Narrative and Counterfactuals in Historical Institutionalism. *World Politics*, 59(3), pp. 341–69.

Celi, C., Guarascio, D. and Somonazzi, A., 2020. A Fragile and Divided European Union Meets Covid-19: Further Disintegration or 'Hamiltonian Moment'? *Journal of Industrial and Business Economics*, 47, pp. 411–24. https://doi.org/10.1007/s40812-020-00165-8.

Collier, D. and Collier, R. B., [1991] 2002. *Shaping the Political Arena Critical Junctures, the Labor Movement and Regime Dynamics in Latin America*. 2nd ed. Notre Dame, IN: University of Notre Dame Press.

Cortell, A. P. and Peterson, S., 1999. Altered states: Explaining Domestic Institutional Change. *British Journal of Political Science*, 29, pp. 177–203.

Cox, P., 2015. From Economic Crisis to Political Crisis in the European Union? *Fondation Jean Monnet pour L'Europe, Debates and Documents Collections*, Issue 3, September 2015.

Cram, L., 1994. The European Commission as a Multi-organization: Social Policy and IT Policy in the EU, *Journal of European Public Policy*, 1(2), pp. 195–217.

Dinan, D., Nugent, N. and Paterson, W. E., 2016. A Multidimensional Crisis. In: D. Dinan, N. Nugent and W. E. Paterson, eds. *The European Union in Crisis*. New York: Red Globe Press, pp. 1–15.

Dyson, K., 2016. Playing for High Stakes: The Eurozone Crisis. In: D. Dinan, N. Nugent, and W. E. Paterson, eds. *The European Union in Crisis*. New York: Red Globe Press, pp. 54–76.

Eurogroup, 2020. *Report on the Comprehensive Economic Policy Response to the COVID-19 Pandemic*. Available at: www.consilium.europa.eu/pt/press/press-releases/2020/04/09/report-on-the-comprehensive-economic-policy-response-to-the-covid-19-pandemic/. [Accessed 27 November 2020].

European Central Bank, 2010. *Financial Stability Review, June*. Available at: www.ecb.europa.eu/pub/pdf/fsr/financialstabilityreview201006en.pdf.

European Commission, 2017. *The EU and the Migration Crisis*. Luxembourg: EU Publications Office.

European Commission, 2020. *Amendment to the Temporary Framework for State Aid Measures to Support the Economy in the Current COVID-19 Outbreak. Communication, Official Journal of the European Union*, C 164, 3–15. Available at: https://eur-lex.europa.eu/legal-content/EN/TXT/PDF/?uri=CELEX:52020XC0513(01)&from=EN. [Accessed 27 November 2020].

European Parliament, 2015. *The Impact of the Crisis on Fundamental Rights Across Member States of the EU. Comparative Analysis, Study for the Libe Committee*. Available at: www.europarl.europa.eu/RegData/etudes/STUD/2015/510021/IPOL_STU(2015)510021_EN.pdf.

Fugita, M. and Hamaguchi, N., 2020. Globalisation and the COVID-19 Pandemic: A Spatial Economic Perspective. *VoxEU, CEPR*. Available at: https://voxeu.org/article/globalisation-and-covid-19-pandemic. [Accessed 3 December 2020].

Gibson, H. D., Palivos, T. and Tavlas, G. S., 2013. *The Crisis in the Euro Area: An Analytical Overview*. Special Conference Paper. Available at: www.bankofgreece.gr/Publications/SCP201328.pdf. [Accessed 10 December 2020].

Herrero, A. G., 2020. The Pandemic Requires a Coordinated Global Economic Response. *Review of European Economic Policy*, 55(2). Available at: www.intereconomics.eu/pdf-download/year/2020/number/2/article/the-pandemic-requires-a-coordinated-global-economic-response-6145.html. [Accessed 16 November 2020].

Keohane, R. O., 1984. *After Hegemony: Cooperation and Discord in the World Political Economy*. Princeton, NJ: Princeton University Press.

Kingdon, J. W., 2003. *Agendas, Alternatives and Public Policies*. 2nd ed. New York: Longman.

Johnson, T., 2020. Ordinary Patterns in an Extraordinary Crisis: How International Relations Make Sense of the COVID-19 Pandemic? *International Organization*, 74 Supplement, pp. E148–68. https://doi.org/10.1017/S0020818320000430.

Monar, J., 2016. Justice and Home Affairs. *Journal of Common Market Studies*, 54(Annual Review), pp. 134–49.

Monnet, J., 1978. *Memoirs* (Translation R. Mayne). Garden City: Doubleday & Company.

Nanopoulos, E. and Vergis, F., 2019. Introduction: The Elephant in the Room: A Tale of Crisis. In E. Nanopoulos and F. Vergis, ed. *The Crisis behind the Eurocrisis: The Eurocrisis as a Multidimensional Systemic Crisis of the EU*. Cambridge: Cambridge University Press, pp. 1–22.

Oosterhof, P. D., 2020. The 2030 Agenda as a Blueprint for a Post-COVID World. *SDG Knowledge Hub, International Institute for Sustainable Development (IISD)*. Available at: http://sdg.iisd.org/commentary/guest-articles/the-2030-agenda-as-blueprint-for-a-post-covid-world/ [Accessed 5 January 2021].

Radjenovic, A., 2019. Reform of the Dublin System, Briefing EU Legislation in Progress. *EPRS – European Parliamentary Research Service*, March. Available at: www.europarl.europa.eu/RegData/etudes/BRIE/2016/586639/EPRS_BRI%282016%29586639_EN.pdf [Accessed 28 November 2020].

Rhinard, M., 2019. The Crisification of Policy-making in the European Union. *Journal of Common Market Studies*, 57(3), pp. 616–33.

Roder, K.-H., 1985. Global Problems A Challenge to Cooperation Between States of Different Social Systems. *International Political Science Review*, 6(1), pp. 35–43.

Schramm, L., 2019. Solidarity – From the Heart or By Force? The Failed German Leadership in the EU's Refugee and Migrant Crisis. *EUI Working Papers 2019/01*. Available at: https://cadmus.eui.eu/bitstream/handle/1814/60349/RSCAS_2019_01.pdf?sequence=1&isAllowed=y. Accessed 21 November 2020.

Staab, A., 2011. *The European Union Explained: Institutions Actors Global Impact*. 2nd ed. Bloomington: Indiana University Press.

Streeck, W. and Thelen, K., 2005. Introduction: Institutional Change in Advanced Political Economies. In W. Streeck and K. Thelen, ed. *Beyond Continuity: Institutional Change in Advanced Political Economies*. Oxford: Oxford University Press, pp. 3–39.

Tosun, J., Wetzel, A. and Zapryanova, G., 2014. The EU in Crisis: Advancing the Debate. *Journal of European Integration*, 36(3), pp. 195–211, DOI: 10.1080/07036337.2014.886401.

World Health Organization, 2020. *Origin of SARS-Cov-2*. 26 March 2020. Available at: https://apps.who.int/iris/bitstream/handle/10665/332197/WHO-2019-nCoV-FAQ-Virus_origin-2020.1-eng.pdf. [Accessed 28 November 2020].

Zeitlin, J., Nicoli, F. and Laffan, B., 2019. Introduction: The European Union beyond the Polycrisis? Integration and Politicization in an Age of Shifting Cleavages. *Journal of European Public Policy*, 26(2), pp. 1–14.

2 Political and institutional analysis of the crisis

2.1 Introduction

The complexity of the EU multi-level governance affects its role as a crisis manager. The EU is a political system on its own since it displays several features that are characteristic of political systems. It has a well-defined set of institutions for collective decision-making and clear rules governing the relations between and within these institutions; citizens direct their inputs to the political system either directly or through intermediaries (such as political parties and interest groups); the outputs of the political system have an impact on economic, social and political dimensions across the whole system; and the process is continuous (Hix, 2007). The limits of EU competences are governed by the principle of conferral: the EU acts only within the limits of the competences that member states have conferred upon it in the treaties (Article 5, Treaty on the European Union).

This chapter pays attention to the politics of the pandemic, both at the supranational and national levels, focusing on the degree of articulation (or disarticulation) between the two. The limited role of the EU in public health policy (supporting competences for the most part) is taken into consideration. How the problem was perceived and defined initially (national versus common) is also relevant for the assessment in the chapter. The purpose of the chapter is to see how well the EU performed as a political actor in the management of the crisis. The focus is on the interaction of national governments and relevant EU institutions (the European Council, the Council, the Commission, the ECB and the EP), notably to find out whether national unilateralism was paradoxical and at the same time detrimental to the EU and to countries themselves.

The following questions are at stake: was the political dimension of the crisis a shortcoming on the comprehensive reaction to the pandemic? Is there a new balance of powers within the institutional system of the EU? In the aftermath of the crisis, do we have more Europe or less Europe? Section 2.2 briefly analyses how a far-off public health problem suddenly 'upgraded' to a major public health crisis in Europe. Section 2.3 zooms in at the very initial stages of the crisis within the EU, assessing the first reactions, mainly at the

DOI: 10.4324/9781003153900-3

national level. Section 2.4 addresses the EU as a crisis manager during the first year of the pandemic, as new dimensions were added to the initial health problem. Section 2.5 assesses change (or the proposal of change) resulting from the response to the pandemic.

2.2 From a far-off health problem to a crisis within Europe

Whereas recent studies and reports point the beginning of the dissemination of the new coronavirus SARs-CoV-2 (the virus responsible for COVID-19) as early as mid-November 2019[1] (House Foreign Affairs Committee, 2020), officially the first human cases of COVID-19 were first reported from Wuhan, China, in December 2019 (World Health Organization, 2020b). Following the report, investigations were undertaken to understand the epidemiology of the new disease as well as to try to identify the original source of the outbreak.[2] The initial investigations concluded that a significant percentage of the initial reported cases (late December 2020 and early January 2021) had a direct link to the Huanan Wholesale Seafood Market in Wuhan city (World Health Organization, 2020b). In the meantime, the disease rapidly spread worldwide. On 13 January 2020, the first COVID-19 case outside China was reported in Thailand and eight days later the first case was confirmed in the United States (House Foreign Affairs Committee, 2020).

In the EU, the first European case was reported from France on 24 January 2020. At that time, the information and knowledge about the new virus was scarce and the response was essentially essayed at the technical level. Early that month (9 January), the Directorate General for Healthy and Food Safety (DG SANTE) opened an alert notification on the Early Warning and Response System (EWRS),[3] allowing member states to share information on response and communication measures. On the same day the European Centre for Disease Prevention and Control (ECDC) published a Threat Assessment Brief where the risk for travellers was considered low, as no indication existed of human-to-human transmission. Although the report considered that the risk of introduction of the virus in the EU was low, it also noted that it 'cannot be excluded' (European Centre for Disease Prevention and Control, 2020a, p. 2). Only eight days later, when the Health Security Committee (HSC)[4] held its first meeting on the novel coronavirus, the ECDC risk assessment changed from low to moderate, since an indication of person-to-person transmission was reported. Between 17 January and 6 February, the HSC held a total six meetings on the new coronavirus.[5] During this short period of time, the rapid transformation of the perception of the degree of threat as regards disease's transmission was noticeable both in the HSC meetings and in the ECDC Rapid Risk Assessments: from 'low risk' to 'high potential impact' of the COVID-19 outbreaks and 'likely' global spread (Health Security Committee, 2020, p. 1). By the end of January, the new disease was declared by the World Health Organisation (WHO) as a 'public health emergency of international concern' (World Health Organisation, 2020a). The perception of threat accelerated in late February and early March and eventually on 11 March 2020 the Director General of the WHO officially declared COVID-19 a global pandemic. By that time, all EU countries were affected,[6] with Italy standing for 58 per cent of the cases reported and 88 per cent of the EU fatalities related to the new disease (European Centre for Disease Prevention and Control, 2020b). In the following days, considering that COVID-19 was 'rapidly spreading worldwide' and that 'the number of cases in Europe… [was] rising in increasing pace in several affected areas' the ECDC called for 'immediate targeted action' (European Centre for Disease Prevention and Control, 2020b, p. 1):

> [a]ll EU/EEA countries should immediately and proactively initiate appropriate, proportional and evidence-based response options to prevent a situation of evolution to scenario 4, where the intensive care capacity is saturated and health systems are overwhelmed.
>
> (European Centre for Disease Prevention and Control, 2020b, p. 8)

As Gaub and Boswinkel noted, although the likelihood of the virus reaching Europe was arguably perceived accurately, 'the lethality and speed of the virus were underestimated both by the media and by decision-makers' (2020, p. 5). For the authors, the pandemic proved that the perception of threat does not necessarily increase at the same pace of the threat itself. It took an increase in fatality rates to attract public awareness of the full severity of the virus and to lead governments to implement strict emergency measures (Gaub and Boswinkel, 2020). One possible explanation is the fact that COVID-19 resembled past crisis trigged by other respiratory diseases such as the severe acute respiratory syndrome (SARS) and the swine flu, which turned out to be a much smaller problem in Europe than what was initially expected. These previous experiences might therefore have lowered the threat perception in European countries in the early stages of COVID-19 spreading (Gaub and Boswinkel, 2020). Pairing the technical monitoring of the threat, an initially tentative and afterwards assertive political response, both at the national and the supranational levels, was implemented, as the following sections illustrate.

2.3 Early national cacophony: the politics of 'everyman for himself'

Shortly after the first reported European case, several member states started to report cases of COVID-19. Yet, Italy was by far the most affected country. Before the end of February, several Italian regions were severely affected, which led the Italian authorities to issue a decree (8 March 2020) to impose strict public health measures including social distancing, which started in the most affected regions and eventually were extended to the whole country (European Centre for Disease Prevention and Control, 2021). Similar public health measures were adopted in many other European countries (European

Centre for Disease Prevention and Control, 2021). Since the disease was new and therefore effective medical countermeasures were nonexistent at that time, national response to COVID-19 was essentially based on non-medical measures (Sabat et al., 2020), which had an impact on different areas, namely freedom of movement (see Chapter 4). Several containment measures were implemented, ranging from lockdowns and travel restrictions to school closures and prohibitions of large gatherings (International Monetary Fund, 2020).

Although the new coronavirus was not initially considered by the EU as an acceptable justification to halt the Schengen Agreement, on 13 March 2020 three member states (Malta, Slovakia and Czech Republic) unilaterally closed borders to Italian citizens and citizens from some other EU member states as a strategy to stop the spread of the disease.[7] Within the Schengen Area between 12 and 19 March, 14 EU member states[8] (and three non-EU member states: Switzerland, Iceland and Norway) notified the Commission about the reintroduction of border controls to reduce the spread of the coronavirus. Although without formally notifying the Commission, also Italy, Slovenia, the Netherlands, Malta and Latvia had in place restrictions on border crossing. The same happened outside the Schengen Area, as of March 2020 all EU member states (except for Ireland) implemented border measures on the grounds of a public health threat (Sabbati and Dumbrava, 2020). However, despite the convergence on the need to adopt circulation limitations, the restrictions adopted by each member state significantly varied as regards the pace, the list of countries whose citizens were temporarily 'banned', as well as the type, severity and length of restrictions, which added to the image of profound discoordination between EU member states.

Another source of division at the initial stage of the public health crisis was the appearance of 'rhetorical clashes' resembling those of the Eurozone crisis. Some controversial public declarations from EU leaders further contributed to the image of disunion and lack of solidarity. One example was Czech Prime Minister Andrej Babis' claim that Italy should ban all its citizens from travelling to the rest of Europe (Reuters, 2020). According to Margalef (2020, p. 1):

> [m]ember states' initial reactions to the coronavirus crisis did not scream solidarity, a value on which the European Union is supposed to be founded. On the contrary, some governments once again reacted by cleaving to austerity as a value and closing borders as a protection measure.

This type of narrative was received with strong frustration by the Southern countries (Margalef, 2020), as neither the pandemic originated in the South nor it was a consequence of Southern member states' actions. The perception of an initial disarray in the response to the COVID-19 crisis can be summed up by the words of Esteban González Pons, a member of the European People's Party group of the EP, during a debate with the President of the Commission: '[f]aced with a single problem, the European member states have given 27 different responses, as if the virus stopped at each border' (Pons quoted in Rios, 2020). The President of the Commission also repeatedly criticised the lack of European solidarity (see section below), and so did the former Commission President, Jacques Delors, who warned against its perils:

> [t]he germ [of division] is back. The climate that seems to hang over the heads of state and government and the lack of European solidarity pose a mortal danger to the European Union.
>
> (Delors, 2020)[9]

Besides the image of lack of solidarity, some member states' actions revealed fierce competitiveness, which initially hampered the EU's ability to respond to the pandemic. Indeed, according to the preliminary results of the HERoS project (which has been assessing the EU early response to COVID-19), the competition between European countries for equipment, test kits and medicines needed to tackle COVID-19 'was all quite counterproductive' (Kovács cited in Gray, 2020). In a similar vein, the so-called vaccine nationalism[10] (during more advanced stages of the pandemic), clearly highlighted the perils of national egoism, not only for the Union as a whole, but for each state's ability to protect its citizens. Fortunately, the EU experienced only glances of 'vaccine nationalism' (see Chapter 5), in part abandoned in favour of a joint procurement by the Commission.

Reflecting on the initial responses of EU member states to the pandemic, Deen and Kruijver consider that those responses, including closing borders, are in line with how normally individual states react to major external threats perceived as security threats:

> (…) the first reflex is one of separation: each European country prioritises the protection of its own population and distancing is an essential part of containing the pandemic.
>
> (Deen and Kruijver, 2020, p. 2)

However, the slow reaction of member states following Italy's request to activate the European Union Civil Protection Mechanism (henceforth Union Mechanism) was striking (Deen and Kruijver, 2020). Indeed, on 26 February, the Italian authorities made a request through the Union Mechanism to get additional personal protective equipment, particularly masks. Even though the Commission activated the Mechanism, no immediate response from the other member states occurred (De Pooter, 2020; Beaucillon, 2020). Actually, some member states (including France and Germany) even banned the export of medical equipment (Gostyńska-Jakubowska and Scazzieri, 2020), although this decision was reverted shortly after. The early silence of the other EU member states casted serious doubts on EU's cohesion and credibility and fuelled the perception amongst Italians and other European citizens that third countries, namely China, helped more than the EU did.

All in all, confronted with an unknown, but rapidly spreading, new disease, national governments have initially taken central stage in the crisis response, but clearly underestimated the importance of coordination and joint communication and action. The absence of articulation hampered the effectiveness of their response and made the perception of European unity fragile. Indeed, it contributed to the construction of an image of profound disunion, largely disseminated by the media worldwide:

> For weeks, the media coverage across Europe was dominated by articles about unilateral border closures, export bans on medical equipment, and the bitter dispute over 'coronabonds'. It is thus unsurprising that many citizens – especially in Italy – were massively disappointed by the crisis management at the European level.
>
> (Loss and Puglierin, 2020)

However, as Loss and Puglierin (2020) noted, although the idea that Europe lacked solidarity at the early stages of the pandemic response was firmly established in European citizens' minds, the reality is more nuanced as a 'dense network of mutual help and cooperation' existed throughout Europe[11] and action taken by EU institutions started early on.

2.4 The central stage for EU institutions: from national unilateralism to European response

Despite the image of incoordination and the sense of disarray highlighted in the section above, the involvement of EU institutions, particularly the Commission, in the management of the pandemic started in the early stages of the crisis. As we noted at the beginning of this chapter, the EU can only act within the limits of the competences conferred to it by the Treaties. In the public health domain, Article 168 of the Treaty on the Functioning of the European Union (TFEU) establishes the bounds of the Union's competences (mostly supporting competences) by stating that the EU action:

> (…) which shall complement national policies, shall be directed towards improving public health, preventing physical and mental illness and diseases, and obviating sources of danger to physical and mental health. Such action shall cover the fight against the major health scourges, by promoting research into their causes, their transmission and their prevention, as well as health information and education, and monitoring, early warning of and combating serious cross-border threats to health.
>
> (Article 168, no 1, TFEU)

However, the same article stipulates that the EU 'shall encourage cooperation between the member states in the areas referred to in this Article and, if necessary, lend support to their action' and entrusts the Commission to 'take any useful initiative to promote such coordination' (Article 168. no 2., TFEU). Additionally, for example, the EU Global Strategy (the strategic document in the field of foreign policy) explicitly states that '[o]n health, we will work for more effective prevention, detection and responses to global pandemics' (European Council/Council of the European Union, 2016, p. 43). What is more, the concerns and action regarding a public health threat encroaches in other policy areas where the Union shares competences with member states, such as freedom of movement and more generally the Single Market (SM). The unfolding of the crisis's multiple layers further widened the areas that fall within the EU shared competences.

As in many other areas, the evolution of the integration process also expanded the possibilities for de facto EU action, even if they are not explicitly enshrined in the treaties. For some decades now, the EU has been enhancing its crisis management capacity. Major developments occur normally as a result of a serious crisis. Indeed, while member states are often reluctant to transfer more authority to the supranational level, they normally call for additional EU capacities to coordinate, link or integrate their response capacities after a large-scale crisis or disaster (Boin, Ekengren and Rhinard, 2013). For example, the idea of creating a crisis response mechanism at the EU level emerged in the early 2000s, triggered by several dramatic events, including the 9/11 attacks (2001), the terrorist attacks in Madrid (2004) and in London (2005) and the tsunami in the Indian Ocean (2004). As a result, in 2006, the Council adopted the emergency and crisis coordination arrangements (CAA), a platform for exchanging information and coordinating action between member states in case of a major crisis. On 25 June 2013, the CAA was substituted by the integrated political crisis response arrangements (IPCR), which added flexibility and scalability to the existing resources, structures and capabilities.[12] On 28 January 2020, the Croatian Presidency of the Council activated the IPCR in information sharing mode (European Council/Council of the European Union, n.d.).

The EU also experienced several previous health crises, such as the BSE epidemic in the early 1990s, the SARS outbreak in 2003 and the 2009 H1N1 influenza pandemic and learned from the shortcomings of its response, namely by adjusting its crisis management structures and procedures. For example, the idea of creating a European public health agency emerged precisely during the SARS outbreak when it became clear that there was a lack of coordination in member states' responses to the outbreak, as well as a need for scientific advice regarding the course of action. The result was the creation of the ECDC in 2005. Another important development, this time following the H1N1 crisis, was the Cross-Border Health Threat Decision (2013),[13] which in practice expanded the EU competences during a public health crisis (Herszenhorn, Paun and Deutsch, 2020), providing a coordinated response leaded by the Commission 'in liaison with the Member States' to public health threats. Equally important was the decision to create the Union Mechanism,[14] which succeeded the Civil Protection Mechanism set up in 2001. The Union Mechanism was used from early stages of the crisis, for example, for the repatriation of European citizens.[15] The H1N1 influenza crisis also exposed weaknesses in the access and purchasing power of EU countries to obtain pandemic vaccines and medications. The Commission was therefore entrusted by the Council to develop a mechanism to jointly procure medical countermeasures that would support fair and equitable access to, and distribution of, pandemic influenza vaccines for the future. The result was the Joint Procurement Agreement (JPA) for medical countermeasures (approved by the Commission in 2014), which enables participating EU countries[16] and the EU institutions to jointly purchase medical countermeasures for different categories of cross-border health threats, including vaccines, antivirals and other treatments (European Commission, n.d.a). The JPA was used during the pandemic crisis to buy personal protective equipment (PPE), as well as COVID-19 vaccines.

Even though there is no doubt that health policy is assigned to the national level, the Treaties, the strategic texts and the consolidation of the EU crisis management capacity opened the door for a relevant role by the EU institutions in this area (although necessarily concerted with member states). The first institution to take central stage was the Commission. After early discrete action, with the Commission acting mostly in the backstage,[17] the institution, headed by President Ursula von der Leyen, gradually played a central coordinator role pushing crisis management in the EU to the political level. Arguably, the stepping up of the Commission was a response to member states' unilateral action. At that time, it was clear that at the initial stage of the crisis the EU had missed the opportunity to play a crucial task in crisis management: sense-making. According to Weick (1988, p. 305), the less appropriate the sense-making directed at a crisis, the more likely the crisis will get out of control. Thus, instrumental to the Commission's goal was its attempt, at least in part successful, of controlling the policy narrative, that is, the 'stories told to persuade key decision makers and their constituents to support specific policy choices' (Mintrom and O'Connor, 2020, p. 208). An important part of the Commission's argument was that uncoordinated action equals ineffectiveness. Member states' uncoordinated action was bluntly criticised by the President of the Commission during a joint press conference with executive vice-presidents Vestager and Dombrovskis to present the economic response to the coronavirus crisis:

> The Single Market has to function. It is not good when Member States take unilateral action. Because it always causes a domino effect. (…) Ultimately, it amounts to reintroducing internal borders at a time when solidarity between Member States is needed. (…) In the last few hours, we have seen travel bans and controls being put in place in a number of Member States. Of course, we all want to protect our citizens from the spread of the virus. So let us look together at how we can do that and how we can do that most effectively.
>
> (von der Leyen, 2020a)

Using a well-known strategy,[18] the Commission played the market card (as the SM is a Commission natural realm) in order to assert its authority and to be able to coordinate member states' actions.

The more the severity and the multidimensionality of the crisis became clear, the more the idea of a coordinated answer became appealing. On 13 February 2020 during an extraordinary Employment, Social Policy, Health and Consumer Affairs (EPSCO) Council meeting, health ministers recalled the importance of cooperation in crisis response and called upon the Commission to facilitate that cooperation (European Council/Council of the European Union, n.d). The call was repeated on a Council's second extraordinary meeting of health ministers that took place on 6 March 2020. Likewise, at the beginning of March 2020, the Croatian Presidency of the Council escalated the IPCR mechanism from information-sharing mode to full activation mode (European Council/Council of the European Union, n.d.), strengthening formal coordination at the EU political level between the Commission, the Council, the European External Action Service, member states affected by the crisis and other relevant EU agencies and experts. The presidencies of the Council that followed (respectively the German and the Portuguese) kept the IPCR mechanism in full mode. The Commission's narrative also consistently repeated the need for urgent action based on solidarity and a coordinated strategy[19]:

> When Europe really needed an 'all for one' spirit, too many initially gave an 'only for me' response (…) But it was not long before some felt the consequences of their own uncoordinated action. This is why over the last few weeks we took exceptional and extraordinary measures to coordinate and enable the action that is needed.
>
> (von der Leyen, 2020b)

One important step was the establishment by the President of the Commission of a new Corona Response Team (CRT)[20] to coordinate the EU response to the pandemic, by bringing together the different strands of action (medical field, mobility and transport and economy). The move paid off, as the Commission became involved in all fronts of the crisis,[21] including the economic dimension, at times even overshading institutions that attract more media attention such as the European Council.

One distinctive feature of crisis situations affecting the EU as a whole is that political decision becomes centralised in the European Council (even if the political agreement is followed by a formal legislative process involving the Council and the EP). In practice this greatly increases European Council's visibility and centrality within the EU system of governance. During the first year of the crisis, as it happened during the Eurozone crisis, the European Council held several extraordinary meetings on the subject,[22] but, interestingly enough, the 'summitisation'[23] effect didn't occur this time. Instead, taking a somewhat backseat position, the heads of state or government of EU countries, during a videoconference on the response to the COVID-19 outbreak (10 March 2020), pushed the Commission further into the centre of the stage by instructing the institution to further step up its response to the coronavirus pandemic and to coordinate member states' actions (Vila Maior and Camisão, 2021). A more 'discrete' intervention of the European Council should not, however, be confused with power loss. Actually, the frequency of the European Council meetings is telling of close monitoring of the work of the Commission by member states.

In the economic dimension of the crisis,[24] the Commission responded promptly to the appeal of the European Council, presenting a continuous flow of proposals to mitigate the socio-economic impact of the crisis that were generally quickly endorsed by the other stakeholders with one noticeable exception. Indeed, the most high-profile proposal to countervail the socio-economic effects of the crisis, but also the one that faced stronger resistance from some member states, was the European Recovery Plan. The task to design a recovery plan was entrusted to the Commission by the European Council in late April 2020. The Commission presented the proposal roughly one month later. A period of tough negotiations followed. Whereas the majority of member states backed the Commission's proposal (including France and Germany, whose leaders presented a similar proposal a few days before), some EU countries strongly opposed the grants part of the plan.

The so-called Frugal Four (Austria, Denmark, Sweden and the Netherlands),[25] led by the Dutch Prime Minister Mark Rutte (Khan, 2020), criticised the increase of the EU budget and called for a recovery plan based on loans, since grants will have to be paid by all EU taxpayers. In a joint open letter to the *Financial Times*, they[26] considered that the 'sound way' to use the money borrowed together in the EU 'is to convert it into loans for those who really need them' and called for 'a realistic level of spending' (Lofven et al., 2020). Rapidly, the shadow of the North–South divide that was hanging over due to the initial perception of EU's lack of solidarity towards Italy gained force. What is more, this divide, as observed during the Eurozone crisis, has superseded arguments about net contributions to the EU budget, to become also about values and culture:

> The current dispute is not primarily about money, but values and culture. The main characteristic of the northern mindset is not frugality. It is a sense of moral superiority derived from the protestant work ethic. All our quarrels about economic policy are subsumed into that.
>
> (Munchau, 2020)

In order to overcome the gridlock in the European leaders, the President of the European Council, Charles Michel, had to intervene. He presented a revised version of the European Multiannual Financial Framework (MFF) and the recovery plan (the so-called negobox). A political agreement was finally reached in the European Council on 21 July 2020. As with the majority of the Commission's proposals, the ambition of the proposed recovery plan was curtailed to accommodate divergent preferences of member states. Also, the 'business as usual' attitude of some member states, even when confronted with a crisis of this magnitude, brought back the shadow of disunion. Yet, the quick adoption by the Council and the EP of the legislative proposals that would follow (see Chapter 3) brought the EU back on track.

Another actor that adopted a proactive stance in this dimension of the crisis was the ECB. After receiving some criticisms for doing less than its US counterpart (the Federal Reserve) to halt the economic effects of the pandemic, the ECB replied swiftly with a 'bold monetary policy response' (Mersch, 2020). One of the most impactful actions was its announcement of a Pandemic Emergency Purchase Programme (PEPP) (see Chapter 3). The willingness of the ECB to be an interventive actor was confirmed by the declarations of its President, Christine Lagarde. Just a few hours after the ECB Governing Council's announcement of the PEPP, Lagarde posted on Twitter: 'Extraordinary times requires extraordinary action. There are no limits to our commitment to the euro' (Lagarde, 2020).[27] The press swiftly compared the bold assertion of the ECB President with the type of statements of her predecessor, Mario Draghi, during the Eurozone crisis:

> Eight minutes after Wednesday midnight in Frankfurt, European Central Bank (ECB) president Christine Lagarde took to Twitter to channel her own version of predecessor Mario Draghi's crisis-era 'whatever it takes to preserve the euro' moment.
>
> (Brennan, 2020)

A parallelism with the ECB's action in the Eurozone crisis was established: 'The ECB statement on doing "everything necessary within its mandate" echoed its former intervention in the sovereign debt crisis' (Rettman, 2020). This type of comparison amplified the expectations regarding the ECB's role in the economic front of the pandemic crisis. Interestingly enough, we would need to go back just a few days to see the opposite picture of Lagarde, and the ECB, in the press:

> [f]acing her first big test after replacing Mario Draghi in November, Lagarde sent the wrong message about the ECB's determination to preserve the eurozone through this crisis, even if she was right to press EU governments for ambitious fiscal action.
>
> (Taylor, 2020)

Actually, Lagarde explicitly refused any resemblance with Draghi by asserting that that she did not seek to be 'whatever it takes, number two' (Lagarde cited in Taylor, 2020). The episode is telling of how volatile the assessment of the actions of the EU institutions is or, for what it's worth, the actions of EU member states, in crisis management, and what is more, how important are not only the actions but also the statements of those actors.

In the health dimension of the crisis, the Commission's involvement started earlier. Initially, its actions were essentially directed to funding research on the coronavirus disease. As of 6 March, the Commission supported 18 projects, involving 151 research teams from across the EU and beyond (European Commission, n.d.c), working on improving preparedness and responses to outbreaks, rapid diagnostic tests, as well as new treatments and new vaccines. Gradually the Commission started to take responsibility for areas where member states were stumbling.

Trying to resolve weaknesses in the access and purchasing power of EU countries to obtain PPE, the Commission launched in 28 February 2020 the first of four joint procurements of PPE together with member states.[28] With the same goal in mind, the Commission created on 19 March 2020 a rescEU stockpile of medical equipment (under the Mechanism) such as ventilators and protective masks to be distributed through the Emergency Response Coordination Centre (ERCC) to the member states that needed more this type of equipment. Both initiatives, along with the first responses to the economic effects of the crisis, paved the way for a change in the narrative, from a disunited to a truly united Europe. The President of the Commission was instrumental to this shift. During the crisis management she revealed crucial communications skills, conveying an image of truth and honesty (Leaders League, 2020). The attention to narrative construction and to the clarity of the communication are crucial assets to frame policy narrative, particularly in times of crisis. Since crisis represents a moment of disruption, there is a need for political leaders to engage in 'meaning-making' (or sense-making), that is, 'providing persuasive accounts of what is happening, why is happening, and what can be done about it' (Mintrom and O'Connor, 2020, p. 209). The President of the Commission embodied this role. She was not afraid to recognise that in the early stages of the crisis the EU was ill-prepared for the pandemic and even offered a 'heartfelt apology' to Italy (von der Leyen, 2020c). But when member states started to collaborate, she also seized every opportunity to highlight examples of Europe's unity, while consistently appealing for a joint approach to tackle the crisis (Leaders League, 2020):

> [t]hough coordination and solidarity between Member States were put into question at the outset of the pandemic, the past few weeks have seen growing examples of solidarity throughout the EU (…).
>
> (von der Leyen and Michel, 2020)

One emblematic action in the health dimension was the EU vaccine strategy (see Chapter 5). Still, the process that culminated with the joint procurement was not without hurdles. In June 2020, Germany, France, followed by Italy and the Netherlands, formed the so-called Inclusive Vaccine Alliance. While the group endorsed the idea of joint procurement, the four countries initiated separate talks with the pharmaceutical industry to buy vaccines and even announced a deal with AstraZeneca, causing discomfort amongst other EU member states, such as Belgium (Deutsch and Wheaton, 2021). Eventually, they decided to step back and opted for the joint procurement (European Commission, 2020c), allowing the Commission to take central stage in the process.

The initiative, although brief, brought to light latent tensions in the EU, reopening the old division between rich and powerful EU countries and poor ones. However, the adoption of the EU vaccine strategy toned down the divisions. Actually, it was a milestone for a shift in the narrative as it highlighted not only the ability but also the willingness of EU member states to cooperate. Unfortunately, this 'unity' started to show some breaches when the actual vaccine campaign in member states began to experience a slow-down in the pace initially established. Criticisms targeting the Commission's action immediately emerged, and the idea that the EU was falling behind made the headlines of the press, fuelling the 'blame game'. Voices calling for individual, national, procurement become louder, and some national leaders accused the Commission's plan of 'being too bureaucratic, too limiting to its members, too slow' (Deutsch and Wheaton, 2021).

The Commission's initial reaction was to threaten AstraZeneca with legal action. EU Health Commissioner Stella Kyriakides bluntly accused the company of breaching contractual obligations and of prioritising the UK over the EU (where AstraZeneca have a vaccine plant). The tensions escalated when AstraZeneca's Chief Executive, Pascal Soriot, rejected the contractual obligation to supply a certain number of doses of the COVID-19 vaccine to the EU, while recalling that the UK made contractual arrangements with AstraZeneca three months before the EU:

> Anyway, we didn't commit with the EU, by the way. It's not a commitment we have to Europe: it's a best effort, we said we are going to make our best effort.
>
> (Soriot cited in Guerrera et al., 2021)

During the dispute, arguably to put pressure on the company, the Commission launched a scheme to monitor the exports of vaccines produced in the EU territory, which required that vaccine exports outside the EU are subject to an authorisation by member states (with the exception of exports under the COVAX). Whereas the scheme was only meant to apply to exports from companies with whom the EU had concluded JPA, the proposal included the possibility of activating Article 16 of the Northern Ireland Protocol (Liboreiro, 2021). After what the media described as 'a flurry of calls between UK and EU leaders,'[29] and an array of criticisms accusing the Commission of betraying its long-time principles (free trade and multilateralism) by resorting to protectionism in the midst of a global health crisis (Liboreiro, 2021), the decision to invoke Article 16 was reversed. Just before transforming into a 'vaccine war' that might have damaged the still very fragile relations with the former EU member (Stevis-Gridneff and Erlanger, 2021), the conflict toned down when AstraZeneca agreed to increase COVID-19 vaccines deliveries to the EU (Hoecklin, 2021). Yet, as the company failed to fulfil its promises, the Commission toughened its position again by proposing to introduce the principles of reciprocity and proportionality as new criteria to be considered to authorise exports under the transparency and authorisation mechanisms for COVID-19 vaccine exports (European Commission, 2021a). This time the escalation of the conflict was avoided by some member states' reluctance to fully back the Commission's tough stance (Dettmer, 2021).

The whole 'vaccine war novel' tainted the image of the Commission and, particularly, that of Ursula von der Leyen, who was accused in the press of troughing the Commission's officials under the bus to save her face (Stevis-Gridneff and Erlanger, 2021). It also negatively affected the Commission's ability to control the policy narrative. As Mintrom and O'Connor noted, no matter how good the narrative is and how engaged the delivery is, if the policies implemented failed to confirm that narrative, then trust and cooperation will wane (2020, p. 218). Meanwhile, other incidents related to COVID-19 vaccines also tested the image of EU's unity, namely bilateral negotiations, first between Hungary and Russia, and afterwards between Slovakia and Russia, to buy the Russian COVID-19 vaccine, Sputnik V. It is true that from a health standpoint, any vaccine that could save lives should be considered. However, the fact that the decision was not taken at the EU level and, what is more, the EU regulator in health matters, the European Medicines Agency, had not yet granted authorisation for Russia's Sputnik V vaccine, hampers not only the EU's image of unity but also the EU's ability to act as a united front towards Russia in times where the diplomatic relations between the two actors are under considerable strain.[30]

On the mobility front,[31] member states were the first to take action. However, it didn't take the Commission too long to intervene, as freedom of movement is the building block of the SM. Indeed, one of the Commission's first documents in this area (issued on 16 March 2020)[32] expressed a clear concern with the SM, namely by proposing measures to ensure that a continuous flow of goods across EU was maintained via green lanes and to ensure the free mobility of critical workers. The Commission also directed its attention to external borders, by recommending the swift adoption by the European Council of a coordinated decision to apply a temporary restriction of non-essential travel from third countries into the EU+ area. The decision was adopted by the European Council in the following day and was successively extended until 15 June 2020.

Meanwhile, in mid-April 2020, the President of the Commission and the President of the European Council presented a *Joint European Roadmap Towards Lifting COVID-19 Containment Measures*. Throughout the document, the imperative of coordinated action was recurrently stressed (coordination-related words feature sixteen times in the document) and was presented as one of the three principles[33] that should guide the EU and member states.

As the first wave of the crisis started to fade, concrete measures to 'reopen' Europe were implemented,[34] including the gradual lift of internal border controls, the reopening of external borders and the restart of economic activity.

Unfortunately, despite the learning process during the first stages of the pandemic and concrete actions to increase the level of preparedness for future outbreaks, the mutation of the virus (towards more aggressive or more easily spread strains) paired with an increase of mobility led to a resurgence of a high number of COVID-19 cases, with member states and the rest of the world experiencing, although at a different pace, the second and third waves of the pandemic. As a result, neither the EU's nor member states' preventing measures were able to avoid new partial or even generalised lockdowns. Although a lack of synchronisation regarding the restrictive measures adopted by member states was also visible during COVID-19 second and third waves, during the first wave this disarticulation resulted more from a lack of communication and coordination, whereas in the second and third waves it is perhaps more due to differences in the beginning of the second and third waves and in the number of casualties directly attributed to COVID-19 in each member state.

All in all, an assessment of the EU's response to the crisis may not grant it a perfect score but does not confirm its allegedly absence:

> Initial knee-jerk competition for scarce medical resources and unilateral actions by Member States in the single market and Schengen Area quickly evolved into improved cooperation and coordination, facilitated by the Commission.
>
> (European Commission, 2020e, p. 6)

The Commission has been consistently active during crisis management. It seems fair to recognise that, although with mixed assessment, the President of the Commission was bold and assertive and made a consistent effort to change the mainstream 'disunion narrative'. The growing prominence of the Commission was well served by von der Leyen's communication skills. Also, the Commission, in collaboration with the other EU institutions, made an important effort to counter disinformation campaigns, the so-called 'infodemic',[35] which contributes to the spread of false narratives, creates confusion and distrust and undermines an effective public health response (European Commission 2020a, p. 1). However, as the would-be 'vaccine war' episode illustrated, in the face of a problem of this magnitude, any false move from one actor can easily undermine the reputation of a policy or the actor itself, even if its performance is not very far from the defined goals.

In the EU institutions interplay, one noticeable 'absence', at least in terms of prominence, was the EP. According to von Ondarza (2020) several reasons might explain this: firstly, times of crisis tend to favour intergovernmental solutions, as decisions need to be quick and the European Council gains visibility; secondly, like its national counterparts, the work of the EP was severely constrained by the pandemic (with the cancellation of plenary sessions in Strasbourg and very limited parliamentary work in Brussels); thirdly, the pandemic has forced the formalisation of the decision-making process and has pushed the EP to work mainly under the 'urgent procedure', which gives the institution less room to propose amendments to the proposals. The limitations were noted by the EP:

> [t]he sudden onset of the COVID-19 pandemic posed a serious challenge to the work of the European Parliament, affecting many activities, official visits, as well as ordinary committee meetings. Therefore, it was essential to prevent the democratic machinery of the EU from potentially coming to a halt.
>
> (European Parliament, 2020, p. 3)

That being said, the EP exercised its scrutinising role during the pandemic, closely following the action of the other institutions, namely the Commission, by holding hearings and exchange views on the management of the pandemics (European Parliament, 2020, p. 4) and by making unusually use of parliamentary questions (von Ondarza, 2020, p. 4). Likewise, the fast-forwarding of the adoption of the proposals was perceived by the EP as a way of contributing for a timely EU response to the pandemic:

> [c]onsidering the seriousness of the situation, a number of the Commission proposals were amended at the Parliament's initiative within a mere 2 to 4 weeks from proposal date to publication.
>
> (European Parliament, 2020, p. 4)

2.5 Assessing change: the proposals to enhance EU preparedness and response capacity

The COVID-19 pandemic showed that a piecemeal approach to a common problem often results in poor, unfitted solutions. As with many other crises, the current pandemic opened a window of opportunity to reform existing policies or to push forward the integration in sectoral areas where the EU has a limited role. As a result of its formal and informal roles, the Commission often seizes these opportunities to put its priorities higher in the European agenda. This policy entrepreneurship is noticeable, for example, in the explicit linkage between the EU Recovery Plan and some of the Commission's pet proposals, such as the Green Deal or a Europe fit for the digital era (two of the von der Leyen's Commission priorities).

One crucial area where weaknesses surfaced is the EU risk governance and crisis management, particularly in areas where member states retain most of their competences. In the first layer of the COVID-19 crisis, the sanitary dimension, crisis response showed that, despite having a legal binding instrument (the 2013 EU Decision on Serious Crossborder Threats to Health) and a dedicated agency (ECDC), the EU health governance framework revealed important shortcomings: early warning and prevention strategies are not sufficiently integrated with responses; limited EU competences on public health hamper efficiency during a pandemic response; and the data shared lacked consistency in terms of quality and level of detail (Renda and Castro, 2021, p. 277). These problems were confirmed by the *2020 Strategic Foresight Report – Charting the Course Towards a More Resilient Europe* produced by the Commission:

> *[t]he COVID-19 crisis has exposed a number of vulnerabilities in the EU and its Member States* (...) Preparedness and prevention, early warning systems and coordination structures were clearly under strain, thus underlining the need for more ambitious crisis management for large-scale emergencies at EU level.
>
> (European Commission, 2020e, p. 5, emphasis in the original)

This less than perfect assessment opened the window of opportunity for introducing change. The Commission took the opportunity. One example was the proposal to build a European Health Union. The idea was put forward by von der Leyen in her first State of the Union address (16 September 2020). Less than two months later, on 11 November, the Commission issued the communication *Building a European Health Union: Reinforcing the EU's Resilience for Cross-border Health Threats*, proposing the 'first building blocks for a European Health Union' (European Commission, 2020d, p. 3). The new Health Union envisioned an upgrade of the EU framework for dealing with cross-border health threats (implemented in 2013) through three new legislative proposals: 'an upgrading of Decision 1082/2013/EU on serious cross-border health threats, a strengthening of the mandate of the European Centre for Disease Prevention and Control (ECDC), and an extension of the mandate of the European Medicines Agency (EMA)' (European Commission, 2020d, p. 3)

Together with a proposal for reinforcing the Union Civil Protection Mechanism (June 2020),[36] the goal was to strengthen EU coordination and resilience, while increasing preparedness both at the EU and the national levels. In the same document, the Commission has also set out the main elements of a new structure – the Health Emergency Response Authority (HERA) – a bio-preparedness authority entrusted with enabling the EU and member states to rapidly deploy most advanced medical and other measures in the event of a health emergency, by covering the whole value chain from conception to distribution and use (European Commission 2020d, p. 20). The initiative, which is currently under public consultation, was preceded by a bio-defence preparedness plan (HERA incubator) designed to facilitate private–public cooperation.

Whereas the new proposals fail to challenge current Treaty provisions as regards public health, therefore maintaining member states' competence in the area, they have the potential to reinforce the EU's capacity to respond to larger-scale emergencies. Beyond the health dimension, the expectation is that 'the lessons learned from these months of lockdown become the foundations of a new approach to risk governance at EU and global levels' (Renda and Castro, 2020, p. 282).

Conclusions

The complexity of the EU political system and variations of EU's competence across policy areas affect its performance as a crisis manager. In this chapter we have looked to the politics of the pandemic, trying to identify the dynamics that shaped the interaction (or the absence of it) between EU institutions and national governments. Our goal was to assess how well the EU performed as a political actor in the management of the crisis.

The tracing of the events suggests that, at the early stages of the pandemic, EU institutions missed the opportunity to set the tone of the response. It was not that EU institutions (particularly the Commission) were absent. But the problem was initially handled by the technical structures. Several factors explain the 'invisibility' of the supranational level. The EU has limited competences in public health policy; at the outset of the crisis there was very limited knowledge of the disease and the information regarding the spread and the consequences of the virus was controlled by Chinese authorities; previous public health crises (such as SARS or H1N1 virus) have turned out to be much less serious in Europe than what was initially anticipated, which might account for an underestimation of the gravity of the novel coronavirus (even by the WHO). Regardless the reasons, the early 'light touch' response was indicative of weaknesses in the EU crisis management capacity, particularly as regarding preparedness.

When EU political leaders finally realised the seriousness of the threat, no EU concerted response to the crisis have been devised; instead, 27 uncoordinated responses were put forward, conveying an image of disunion, lack of solidarity and helpless Europe. At this point, between press headlines praising China's 'generosity' for helping Italy and analysts predicting the end of the European project, the odds were for less Europe in the aftermath of the pandemic. However, it didn't take the Commission too long to reassert its role as coordinator of the EU response to the crisis, first using the SM entryway, and afterwards due to the general acceptance that this was the role the Commission should play.

The ECB also rose to the challenge by presenting assertive responses to the crisis, whereas the European Council, a more 'natural' leader (considering the experience of previous crises) adopted (at least initially) a lower profile, although meeting frequently. Does this mean that there is a new balance of powers within the institutional system of the EU? Our findings suggest that, despite the prominence of the Commission (that confirms the path initiated in the Juncker Commission towards regaining centrality), the institutional balance was not fundamentally altered. The EU response is still in part shaped by intergovernmental bargaining. The EP, although this time for justifiable reasons, seems to continue a trend of less visibility (despite its crucial role as co-legislator), perhaps due to the 'crisification' (Rhinard, 2019) of European policymaking.

As many others before it, the pandemic crisis opened a window of opportunity for reform. The consciousness of the limitations in terms of preparedness and prevention at the EU level triggered several proposals for reform in the policy areas affected by the pandemic, particularly health policy. Although not suggesting radical change, if adopted, these proposals could represent an important push forward, resulting in more Europe.

Notes

1 Despite some consensus around December as the month of the outbreak, the search for 'patient zero' remains active.

2 In January 2021 a joint international team comprising 17 Chinese and 17 international experts from other countries, the WHO, the Global Outbreak Alert and Response Network (GOARN) and the World Organisation for Animal Health conducted a joint study probing the origin of the COVID-19 pandemic, over a 28-day period (from 14 January to 10 February 2021) in the city of Wuhan, People's Republic of China. BBC news. 'Covid: WHO Team Probing Origin of Virus Arrives at China'. Available at: www.bbc.com/news/world-asia-china-55657781 [Accessed 28 January 2021]. The report of the international team was published on 30 March 2021. The joint team of experts examined the likelihood of four scenarios: direct zoonotic transmission to humans (possible-to-likely pathway); introduction through an intermediate host followed by spillover (likely to very likely pathway); introduction through the (cold) food chain (possible pathway); and introduction through a laboratory incident (extremely unlikely pathway). However, no definitive conclusions were presented regarding the origins of the virus. Instead, the report called for further investigation (World Health Organization, 2021, p. 9).

3 The EWRS is a tool for monitoring health threats in the EU. The access to and posting of information is restricted to the European Centre for Disease Control (ECDC), member states and DG SANTE. See European Centre For Disease Control webpage. Available online at: www.ecdc.europa.eu/en/publications-data/early-warning-and-response-system-european-union-ewrs [Accessed 29 December 2020].

4 The HSC is an informal advisory group on health security at the EU level set up in 2001 at the request of EU health ministers. In 2013 its mandate was formalised and strengthened (Decision 1082/2013/EU), making the Committee in charge of reinforcing the coordination and sharing of best practice and information on national preparedness activities. Within the Committee, member states consult each other in order to coordinate national responses to serious cross-border threats to health. The HSC is chaired by a representative of the Commission, which also provides the secretariat. See European Commission, Health Security and Infectious Diseases webpage. Available online at: https://ec.europa.eu/health/preparedness_response/risk_management/hsc/members_pt [Accessed 29 December 2020].

5 The meetings took place on the 17, 22, 27, 31 January and on 4 and 6 February.

6 According to the ECDC, a total of 17,413 cases were reported as of 11 March 2020.

7 See ShengenVisaInformation.com, Schengen Area Crisis: EU States Close Borders as Coronavirus Outbreak Grips Bloc, 13 March 2020. Available at: www.schengenvisainfo.com/news/schengen-area-crisis-eu-states-close-borders-as-coronavirus-outbreak-grips-bloc/ [Accessed 4 January 2021].

8 Belgium, Czechia, Denmark, Germany, Estonia, Spain, France, Lithuania, Hungary, Austria, Poland, Portugal, Slovakia and Finland.

9 Delors cited in Agence France Press. 'Epidemic Infects Europe with "Germ of Division'". 28 March 2020. Available at: www.france24.com/en/20200328-epidemic-infects-europe-with-germ-of-division [Accessed 11 January 2021].

10 Here we use the concept of 'vaccine nationalism' in a narrow sense, to describe the actions of some EU member states that were more concerned to guarantee vaccination for its own citizens, than to secure the protection of all EU citizens. However, there is a broader, more relevant, debate that highlights the differences worldwide, notably between the industrialized North and the underdeveloped South. The debate revolves around the idea that leaders of the wealthier countries are prioritising their own countries over the planet. Indeed, richest countries are buying a big part of vaccine production (enough to protect their own population several times over), leaving developing economies struggling to access supplies, as the rhythm of production does not follow the rhythm of demand and prices are spiking exponentially.

11 See for example European Solidarity Tracker, a project by the European Council on Foreign Relations that 'collects and displays instances of pan-European solidarity throughout the coronavirus crisis'. Available at: https://ecfr.eu/special/solidaritytracker/ [Accessed 28 January 2021].

12 The IPCR aim is to strengthen the EU's ability to take rapid decisions when facing major cross-sectoral crises requiring a response at EU political level, by providing the necessary support from EU institutions and services in the context of a crisis and its evolution (European Council/Council of the European Union, 2020). In 2018 it was codified into a legal act through a Council implementing decision (European Council/Council of the European Union, n.d.). See Council Implementing Decision (EU) 2018/1993 of 11 December 2018 on the EU Integrated Political Crisis Response Arrangements. Available at: https://eur-lex.europa.eu/legal-content/EN/TXT/PDF/?uri=CELEX:32018D1993&qid=1583154099617&from=EN [Accessed 2 February 2021].

13 Decision No 1082/2013/EU of the European Parliament and of the Council of 22 October 2013 on serious cross-border threats to health and repealing Decision No 2119/98/EC. Available at: https://eur-lex.europa.eu/legal-content/EN/TXT/PDF/?uri=CELEX:32013D1082&from=EN [Accessed 11 January 2021].

14 Decision No. 1313/2013/EU of the European Parliament and of the Council of 17 December 2013 on a Union Civil Protection Mechanism, amended by Regulation (EU) 2018/1475 of the European Parliament and of the Council of 2 October 2018 and by Decision (EU) 2019/420 of the European Parliament and of the Council of 13 March 2019.

15 According to the Commission, as of 27 March 2020, more than 10.000 EU citizens were repatriated in flights organized through the Mechanism. See European Commission. Timeline of EU Action. Available at: https://ec.europa.eu/info/live-work-travel-eu/coronavirus-response/timeline-eu-action_en [Accessed 2 February 2021].

16 As of April 2020, the JPA has been signed by 37 countries including all EU and EEA countries, the UK, Albania, Montenegro, North Macedonia, Serbia and Bosnia and Herzegovina, as well as Kosovo (European Commission, n.d.a).

17 Between January and February 2020, some EU level action occurred with the involvement of the Commission, including repatriation of EU citizens, the mobilisation of funds for research on the new coronavirus outbreak, the delivery of PPE to China, the launch of the first of four joint procurements of PPE with member states and giving support to the national authorities.

18 See for example (Brandão and Camisão, 2021).

19 Eventually, the call for coordination echoed within but also outside the EU. For example, on 3 May 2020, an op-ed co-authored by Giuseppe Conte, President of Italy; Emmanuel Macron, President of France; Angela Merkel, Chancellor of Germany; Charles Michel, President of the European Council; Erna Solberg, Prime Minister of Norway; Justin Trudeau, Prime Minister of Canada; and Ursula von der Leyen, President of the Commission, acknowledged that '[n]one of us is immune to the pandemic and none of us can beat the virus alone', therefore highlighting the absolute need for coordination: 'We are building on the commitment by G20 leaders to develop a massive and coordinated response to the virus (…)'. The article also explicitly referred the Access to COVID-19 Tools (ACT) Accelerator, a global cooperation platform created to accelerate and scale-up research, development, access and equitable distribution of the vaccine and other life-saving therapeutics and diagnostics treatments. For the signatories of the op-ed this tool 'laid the foundation for a real international alliance to fight COVID-19'. See, European Commission. 2021. Global Response: Working Together to help the world get better. Available at: https://ec.europa.eu/commission/presscorner/detail/en/AC_20_795 [Accessed 15 April 2021]. On 30 March 2021, 24 world leaders (including some EU leaders such as Germany Chancellor Angela Merkel, France President Emmanuel Macron, Portugal Prime Minister António Costa, the President of the European Council Charles Michel, but also the UK Prime Minister Boris Johnson and the head of the WHO, Tedros Adhanom Ghebreyesus), in an op-ed article, published in several newspapers called for a new global settlement (an international treaty) to enhance the world's preparedness to face future pandemics. See BBC News. COVID-19 World leaders call for international pandemic treaty. Available at: www.bbc.com/news/uk-56572775 [Accessed 15 April 2021]. The op-ed article is available at: www.consilium.europa.eu/en/press/press-releases/2021/03/30/pandemic-treaty-op-ed/ [Accessed 15 April 2021].

20 Five commissioners integrate the CRT: Janez Lenarčič (crisis' management); Stella Kyriakides (health issues); Ylva Johansson (border-related issues); Adina Vălean (mobility); and Paolo Gentiloni (macroeconomic issues).

21 For a detailed timeline of the EU action see, for example, European Commission. (n.d.c) Timeline of EU Action. Available at: https://ec.europa.eu/info/live-work-travel-eu/coronavirus-response/timeline-eu-action_en [Accessed 2 February 2021].

22 According to the dispositions of the Treaty on the European Union (TEU), the European Council 'shall meet twice every six months (…) When the situation so requires, the President shall convene a special meeting of the European Council' (Article 15, No 3, TEU). Between March 2020 and March 2021, the European Council held 15 meetings (including several videoconference meetings to follow the progress of the European response to the COVID-19 outbreak), of which fourteen had the COVID-19 pandemic issue (directly or indirectly) in the agenda.

See, European Council/Council of the European Union. n.d. Meeting calendar. Available at: www.consilium.europa.eu/en/meetings/calendar/?Category=meeting&Page=1&dateFrom=2020%2F03%2F01&dateTo=2021%2F03%2F31&filters=2031 [Accessed 1 April 2021].

23 'Summitisation' was a term coined by Martin Schulz (at the time President of the European Parliament) to criticise the excessive role of the European Council during the Eurozone crisis. In that period, the European Council held an unprecedented number of meetings, capturing media attention and pushing the institution to the centre of EU governance (Dinan, 2013).

24 For more detailed insight on the measures adopted at the EU level to respond to the economic dimension of the crisis, see Chapter 3.

25 The group gained its name during the negotiations of the EU Multiannual Financial Framework (MFF) for 2021–2027, where the block defended a ceiling of 1 per cent of the EU gross national income to the EU budget.

26 The letter was written by the Prime Minister of Sweden, Stefan Lofven, and co-authored by the Prime Ministers of Denmark, Mette Frederiksen, and the Netherlands, Mark Rutte, and the Chancellor of Austria, Sebastian Kurz.

27 See Christine Lagarde on Twitter. Available at: https://twitter.com/lagarde/status/1240414918966480896 [Accessed 2 February 2020].

28 The other three took place on 17 March 2020 (two calls) and on 19 March 2020.

29 Sky News. 'What is Article 16 and Why Did the EU Make a U-turn After Triggering It?" 31 January 2021. Available at: https://news.sky.com/story/what-is-article-16-and-why-did-the-eu-make-a-u-turn-after-triggering-it-12202915 [Accessed 25 February 2021].

30 After a recent trip to Russia, the Head of EU diplomacy, Josep Borrell, said that it became clear that 'Russian authorities did not want to seize this opportunity to have a more constructive dialogue with the EU' and therefore '[a]s EU, we will have to draw the consequences, reflect carefully on the direction we want to give to our relations with Russia and proceed in a united manner with determination' (Borrell, 2021).

31 For a detailed insight on the effects of closing of borders and imposing restrictions to freedom of movement, see Chapter 4.

32 See European Commission, 2020. COVID-19 Guidelines for Border Management Measures to Protect Health and Ensure the Availability of Goods And Essential Services, C(2020) 1753, 16 March 202. Available at: https://eur-lex.europa.eu/legal-content/EN/TXT/PDF/?uri=CELEX:52020XC0316(03)&from=EN [Accessed 8 February 2021].

33 The other two are to base action on science and to have public health at its centre, and the importance of respect and solidarity between member states (von der Leyen and Michel, 2020, p. 6).

34 On 15 June the European Commission launched a web platform dubbed Re-open EU which provides an overview of the health situation in EU countries, based on data from the ECDC. See European Union, Re-open EU. Available at: https://reopen.europa.eu/en/ [Accessed 8 February 2021].

35 The term was coined by the WHO to describe 'an excessive amount of information about a problem, which makes it difficult to identify a solution. They can spread misinformation, disinformation and rumours during a health emergency. Infodemics can hamper an effective public health response and create confusion and distrust among people' (WHO cited in European Commission, 2020c).

36 See European Commission (2020) Proposal for a Decision of the European Parliament and of the Council amending Decision No 1313/2013/EU on a Union Civil Protection Mechanism, COM(2020) 220 final, 2 June 2020. Available at: https://ec.europa.eu/echo/sites/echo-site/files/com_2020_220_en_act_v13.pdf [Accessed 1 March 2021]. The EP and the Council reached agreement on the Commission's proposal on 8 February 2021.

Bibliography

Beaucillon, C., 2020. International and European Emergency Assistance to EU Member States in the COVID-19 Crisis: Why European Solidarity Is Not Dead and What We Need to Make It Both Happen and Last. *European Papers*, 5(1), pp. 387–401. Available at: www.europeanpapers.eu/en/system/files/pdf_version/EP_EF_2020_I_013_Charlotte_Beaucillon.pdf [Accessed 27 November 2020].

Boin, A., Ekengren, M., and Rhinard, M., 2013. *The European Union as Crisis Manager*. Cambridge: Cambridge University Press.

Borrell, J., 2021. My visit to Moscow and the future of EU-Russia relations. HP/VP Blog, 7 February 2021. Available at: https://eeas.europa.eu/headquarters/headquarters-homepage/92722/my-visit-moscow-and-future-eu-russia-relations_en [Accessed 1 March 2021.]

Brandão, A. P., and Camisão, I., 2021. Playing the Market Card: The Commission's Strategy to Shape EU Cybersecurity Strategy. *Journal of Common Market Studies*, pp. 1–21, DOI: 10.1111/jcms.13158.

Brennan, J., 2020. How Lagarde's Flippancy Led to Godsend for EU Governments Fighting Covid-19. *The Irish Times*, 20 March 2020. Available at: www.irishtimes.com/business/how-lagarde-s-flippancy-led-to-godsend-for-eu-governments-fighting-covid-19-1.4208072 [Accessed: 25 February 2021].

De Pooter, H., 2020. The Civil Protection Mechanism of the European Union: A Solidarity Tool at Test by the COVID-19 Pandemic. *American Society of International Law*, 24(7). Available at: www.asil.org/insights/volume/24/issue/7/civil-protection-mechanism-european-union-solidarity-tool-test-covid-19 [Accessed 12 January 2021].

Deen, B. and Kruijver, K., 2020. Corona: EU's Existential Crisis: Why the Lack of Solidarity Threatens Not Only the Union's Health and Economy, But Also Its Security. *Clingendael Alert*, April 2020. Available at: www.clingendael.org/sites/default/files/2020-04/Alert_Corona_Existential_Crisis_April_2020.pdf. [Accessed 11 January 2021].

Dettmer, J. 2021. EU Backs Off Sparking Vaccine War. Voanews, 26 March 2021. Available at: www.voanews.com/covid-19-pandemic/eu-backs-sparking-vaccine-war [Accessed 5 April 2021].

Deutsch, J. and Wheaton, S., 2021. How Europe Fell Behind on Vaccines. *Politico*, 27 January 2021. Available at: www.politico.eu/article/europe-coronavirus-vaccine-struggle-pfizer-biontech-astrazeneca/. [Accessed 16 February 2020].

Dinan, D., 2013. EU Governance and Institutions. *Journal of Common Market Studies*, 51(Annual Review), pp. 89–102.

European Centre for Disease Prevention and Control, 2020a. *Threat Assessment Brief: Pneumonia Cases Possibly Associated with a Novel Coronavirus in Wuhan, China*, 9 January 2020. Available at: www.ecdc.europa.eu/sites/default/files/documents/Threat-assessment-Pneumonia-cases-possibly-associated-to-a-novel-coronavirus-in-Wuhan-China.pdf. [Accessed 27 November 2020].

European Centre for Disease Prevention and Control, 2020b. *Rapid Risk Assessment: Novel Coronavirus Disease 2019 (COVID-19) Pandemic Increased Transmission in the EU/EEA and the UK – Sixth Update 12 March 2020*. Available at: www.ecdc.europa.eu/sites/default/files/documents/RRA-sixth-update-Outbreak-of-novel-coronavirus-disease-2019-COVID-19.pdf. [Accessed 16 December 2020].

European Centre for Disease Prevention and Control, 2021. *Timeline of ECDC's Response to COVID-19*. Available at: www.ecdc.europa.eu/en/covid-19/timeline-ecdc-response. [Accessed 4 March 2021].

European Commission, n.d.a. *Health Security and Infectious Diseases*. Available at: https://ec.europa.eu/health/security/preparedness_response_en. [Accessed 27 November 2020].

European Commission, n.d.c. *Timeline of EU Action*. Available at: https://ec.europa.eu/info/live-work-travel-eu/coronavirus-response/timeline-eu-action_en. [Accessed 27 November 2020].

European Commission, 2020a. *Europe's Moment: Repair and Prepare for the Next Generation*. COM(2020) 456 final. Available at: https://eur-lex.europa.eu/legal-content/EN/TXT/PDF/?uri=CELEX:52020DC0456&from=EN [Accessed 24 November 2020].

European Commission, 2020b. *Tackling COVID-19 Disinformation: Getting the Facts Right*. COM(2020) 8 final, 10 June 2020. Available at: https://eur-lex.europa.eu/legal-content/EN/TXT/PDF/?uri=CELEX:52020JC0008&from=EN. [Accessed 4 December 2020].

European Commission, 2020c. *Coronavirus: The Commission Signs First Contract with AstraZeneca*. Press Release, 27 July 2020. Available at: https://ec.europa.eu/commission/presscorner/detail/en/IP_20_1524. [Accessed 20 November 2020].

European Commission, 2020d. *Building a European Health Union: Reinforcing the EU's Resilience for Cross-border Health Threats*. COM(2020) 724 final, 11 November 2020. Available at: https://eur-lex.europa.eu/legal-content/EN/TXT/PDF/?uri=CELEX:52020DC0724&from=EN. [Accessed 28 November 2020].

European Commission, 2020e. *2020 Strategic Foresight Report – Charting the Course Towards a more Resilient Europe*. Available at: https://ec.europa.eu/info/sites/info/files/strategic_foresight_report_2020_1.pdf. [Accessed 27 November 2020].

European Council/Council of the European Union. n.d. The Council's Response to Crisis (IPCR). Available at: www.consilium.europa.eu/en/policies/ipcr-response-to-crises/. [Accessed 11 January 2021].

European Council/Council of the European Union, 2016. A Global Strategy for the European Union's Foreign and Security Policy. Available at: https://eeas.europa.eu/sites/default/files/eugs_review_web_0.pdf [Accessed 11 January 2021].

European Parliament, 2020. *The European Parliamentary Committees' Response to COVID-19: Ensuring the Continuation of the Legislative and Democratic Life of the European Union An overview*, June 2020. Available at: www.europarl.europa.eu/cmsdata/210129/Committee-activities-COVID19-Full%20document-Final.pdf [Accessed 7 April 2021].

Gaub, F. and Boswinkel, L., 2020. *Who's First Wins: International Crisis Response to COVID-19. European Union Institute for Security Studies*. Brief 11, May 2020. Available at: www.iss.europa.eu/content/who's-first-wins-international-crisis-response-covid-19. [Accessed 3 November 2020].

Gostyńska-Jakubowska, A. and Scazzieri, L., 2020. The EU Needs To Step Up Its Response to the COVID-19 Outbreak. *Centre for European Reform Insight*, 23 March 2020. Available at: www.cer.eu/sites/default/files/insight_AG_LS_23.3.20.pdf. [Accessed 25 November 2020].

Gray, R., 2020. Lack of Solidarity Hampered Europe's Coronavirus Response, Research Finds. *Horizon: The EU Research & Innovation Magazine*. Available at: https://horizon-magazine.eu/article/lack-solidarity-hampered-europe-s-coronavirus-response-research-finds.html. [Accessed 12 December 2020].

Guerrera, A., Bolzen, S. and Miguel, R., 2021. Interview with Pascal Soriot. *La Repubblica*, 26 January 2021. Available at: www.repubblica.it/cronaca/2021/01/26/news/interview_pascal_soriot_ceo_astrazeneca_coronavirus_covid_vaccines-284349628/. [Accessed 5 February 2021].

Health Security Committee, 2020. *Summary: The Cluster of Pneumonia Cases Associated with Novel Coronavirus in Wuhan, China*, 22 January 2020. Available at: https://ec.europa.eu/health/sites/health/files/preparedness_response/docs/ev_20200122_sr_en.pdf. [Accessed 26 November 2020].

Herszenhorn, D. M., Paun, C. and Deutsch, J., 2020. Europe Fails to Help Italy in Coronavirus Fight. *Politico*. Available at: www.politico.eu/article/eu-aims-better-control-coronavirus-responses/. [Accessed 22 November 2020].

Hix, S., 2007. The EU as a New Political System. In: D. Caramani, ed. *Comparative Politics*. Oxford: Oxford University Press, pp. 573–601.

Hoecklin, M., 2021. European Commission Resolves Dispute with AstraZeneca over Covid Vaccine Deliveries – EU Officials Predict More Stable Supplies by April. *Health Policy Watch*, 1 February 2021. Available at: https://healthpolicy-watch.news/european-union-resolves-dispute-with-astrazeneca-over-covid-vaccine-deliveries-eu-officials-predict-more-steady-supplies-by-aprill/. [Accessed 19 February 2021].

House Foreign Affairs Committee, 2020. The Origins of the COVID-19 Global Pandemic, including the Roles of the Chinese Communist Party and the World Health Organization. *House Foreign Affairs Committee Minority Staff Report*. Available at: https://gop-foreignaffairs.house.gov/wp-content/uploads/2020/09/Final-Minority-Report-on-the-Origins-of-the-COVID-19-Global-Pandemic-Including-the-Roles-of-the-CCP-and-WHO-9.20.20-Coverpage.pdf. [Accessed 28 December 2020].

International Monetary Fund, 2020. *Policy Responses to COVID-19*. Available at: www.imf.org/en/Topics/imf-and-covid19/Policy-Responses-to-COVID-19#top. [Accessed 28 November 2020].

Khan, M., 2020. 'Frugal Four' Chief Mark Rutte Leads Opposition to EU Recovery Plan. *Financial Times*, 18 June 2020. Available at: www.ft.com/content/8e30fd89-4958-491e-9f30-8c0b5f8b4cef. [Accessed 27 November 2020].

Leaders League, 2020. *Heroes and Zeros: Ursula von der Leyen The Level-headed One*. Available at: www.leadersleague.com/en/news/heroes-zeros-ursula-von-der-leyen. [Accessed 28 November 2020].

Liboreiro, J., 2021. '*Wholly Unnecessary*'*: Criticism Mounts on Brussels over Vaccine Furore*. 2 February 2021. Available at: www.euronews.com/2021/02/01/wholly-unnecessary-criticism-mounts-on-brussels-over-vaccine-furore. [Accessed 5 March 2021].

Lofven, S., Frederiksen, M., Rutte, M. and Kurz, S., 2020. Open Letter. *Financial Times*, 16 June 2020. Available at: www.ft.com/content/7c47fa9d-6d54-4bde-a1da-2c407a52e471 [Accessed 2 February 2021].

Loss, R. and Puglierin, J., 2020. The Truth about European Solidarity during Corona. European Council on Foreign Relations. *Commentary*, 26 June 2020. Available at: https://ecfr.eu/article/commentary_the_truth_about_european_solidarity_during_corona/. [Accessed 15 December 2020].

Margalef, H. S., 2020. Solidarity and Coronavirus: The End of Naïve Europeanism? *CIDOB Opinion*, May 2020.

Mersch, Y., 2020. *Keynote Speech: Legal aspects of the ECB's Response to the Coronavirus (COVID-19) Pandemic – An Exclusive But Narrow Competence*. Available at: www.ecb.europa.eu/press/key/date/2020/html/ecb.sp201102~5660377b52.en.html. [Accessed 27 November 2020].

Mintrom, M., and O'Connor, R., 2020. The Importance of Policy Narrative: Effective Government Responses to Covid-19. *Policy Design and Practice*, 3(3), pp. 205–27.

Munchau, W., 2020. North versus South. The North South Divide Is Now the Biggest Threat to the EU. It's about Culture More Than Economics. *Euro Intelligence*, October 2020. Available at: www.eurointelligence.com/column/north-and-south [Accessed 5 February 2021].

Renda, A. and Castro, R., 2020. Towards Stronger EU Governance after the COVID-19 Pandemic. *European Journal of Risk Regulation*, 11 (2020), pp. 273–82.

Rettman, A., 2020. ECB Promises (Almost) Whatever It Takes. *euobserver*, 19 March 2020. Available at: https://euobserver.com/coronavirus/147808 [Accessed 25 February 2021].

Reuters, 2020. Czech PM Says Italy Should Ban All Citizens from Travelling to Europe. Available at: https://fr.reuters.com/article/uk-health-coronavirus-czech-italy-idUKKBN20V0BT [Accessed 4 January 2021].

Rhinard, M., 2019. The Crisification of Policy-making in the European Union. *Journal of Common Market Studies*, 57(3), pp. 616–33.

Rios, B., 2020. Commission Chief, MEPs Slam Lack of EU Solidarity in COVID19 crisis, *EURACTIVE.com*, 26 March 2020. Available at: www.euractiv.com/section/coronavirus/news/commission-chief-meps-slam-lack-of-eu-solidarity-in-covid19-crisis/ [Accessed 4 January 2021].

Sabat, I., Neuman-Bhome, S., Varghese, N. E., Barros, P. P, Brouwer, W., van Exel, J., Schreyogg, J. and Stargardt, T., 2020. United but Divided: Policy Responses and People's Perceptions in the EU during the COVID-19 Outbreak. *Health Policy*, 124, pp. 909–18.

Sabbati, G. and Dumbrava, C., 2020. The Impact of Coronavirus on Schengen Borders. *EPRS – European Parliamentary Research Service*, March 2020. Available at: www.europarl.europa.eu/RegData/etudes/BRIE/2020/649347/EPRS_BRI(2020)649347_EN.pdf [Accessed 28 January 2021].

Stevis-Gridneff, M. and Erlanger, S., 2021. The E.U. Official Came Under Fire in Vaccine Wars. *The New York Times*, 1 February 2021. Available at: www.nytimes.com/2021/02/01/world/europe/eu-vaccine-von-der-leyen.html [Accessed 25 February 2021].

Taylor, P., 2020. Lagarde's Corono Blunder. *Politico*, 13 March 2020. Available at: www.politico.eu/article/christine-lagarde-corona-blunder-ecb/ [Accessed 25 February 2021].

Vila Maior, P. and Camisão, I., 2021. Institutional Rebalancing in the Wake of the Covid-19 Pandemic. In: J. Caetano, I. Vieira and A. Caleiro, A., ed. *New Challenges for the Eurozone Governance: Joint Solutions for Common Threats*? Cham: Springer, pp. 285–302.

Von der Leyen, U., 2020a. Remarks by President von der Leyen at the joint press conference with Executive Vice-Presidents Vestager and Dombrovskis to present the economic response to the Coronavirus crisis. 13 March 2020. Available at: https://ec.europa.eu/commission/presscorner/detail/pt/statement_20_465 [Accessed 4 January 2021].

Von der Leyen, U., 2020b. Speech by President von der Leyen at the European Parliament Plenary on the European coordinated response to the COVID-19 outbreak. 26 March 2020. Available at: https://ec.europa.eu/commission/presscorner/detail/en/speech_20_532 [Accessed 4 January 2021].

Von der Leyen, U., 2020c. Speech by President von der Leyen at the European Parliament Plenary on the EU coordinate action to combat the coronavirus pandemic and its consequences. 16 April 2020. Available at: https://ec.europa.eu/commission/presscorner/detail/en/SPEECH_20_675 [Accessed 4 February 2021].

Von der Leyen, U. and Michel, C., 2020. Joint European Roadmap Towards Lifting COVID-19 Containment Measures. 15 April 2020. Available at: https://op.europa.eu/en/publication-detail/-/publication/14188cd6-809f-11ea-bf12-01aa75ed71a1/language-en [Accessed 8 February 2021].

Von Ondarza, N., 2020. The European Parliament's Involvement in the EU Response to the Corona Pandemic. A Spectator in Times of Crisis. *SWP Comment*, No 45 October 2020. Available at: www.swp-berlin.org/fileadmin/contents/products/comments/2020C45_EuropeanParliament.pdf [Accessed 16 February 2021].

Weick, K. E. (1988) Enacted Sensemaking in Crisis Situations. *Journal of Management Studies*, 25(4), pp. 305–317. Available at: https://onlinelibrary.wiley.com/doi/epdf/10.1111/j.1467-6486.1988.tb00039.x. [Accessed 16 February 2021].

World Health Organization, 2020a. Statement on the second meeting of the International Health Regulations (2005) Emergency Committee regarding the outbreak of novel coronavirus (2019-nCoV). 30 January 2020. Available at: www.who.int/news/item/30-01-2020-statement-on-the-second-meeting-of-the-international-health-regulations-(2005)-emergency-committee-regarding-the-outbreak-of-novel-coronavirus-(2019-ncov) [Accessed 4 January 2021].

World Health Organization, 2020b. Origin of SARS-Cov-2. 26 March 2020. Available at: https://apps.who.int/iris/bitstream/handle/10665/332197/WHO-2019-nCoV-FAQ-Virus_origin-2020.1-eng.pdf. [Accessed 28 November 2020].

3 An economic analysis of the pandemic crisis

3.1 Introduction

The pandemic crisis began as a sanitary crisis. Notwithstanding, the several ramifications of the crisis soon started to emerge. Citizens became aware that the crisis was not restricted to the public health dimension and that other areas would also be affected. The economy was squeezed within a short period of time. The pandemic crisis rapidly exposed the challenges to the economy, notably after countries decided to resort to lockdown and many economic activities were shut down. Consequently, government intervention was required to support economic sectors facing the threat of collapse and to prevent workers' loss of income. At the same time, the pandemic crisis had consequences on the economy after governments realised that they should provide massive support to national healthcare systems.

This chapter addresses the economic challenges stemming from the pandemic crisis. It emphasises how a deep economic crisis came after countries were affected not only by the quick spread of COVID-19 but also by severe contingency measures aiming at stopping the contagion of the virus. To this extent, several economic dimensions deserve attention. One is the sudden and severe economic slowdown after governments decided to impose a lockdown on populations and corporations. Section 3.2 collects statistical data on the early estimations of negative economic growth. More importantly, paying attention to comparisons between countries is to engage on an intertemporal analysis that reveals to what extent economic activity suffered losses following governments' strategy against the pandemic. In addition, data on inflation and, especially, on unemployment are needed to corroborate countries' macroeconomic performance as they were impacted by the seismic waves of the pandemic crisis.

Section 3.3 looks at how fiscal policy deteriorated as a mirror of governments' strategies to avoid the massive spread of the virus and to prevent the economy from suffering further damages. Governments' intervention was unprecedented, at least when compared with previous episodes of economic crisis. True, this crisis started outside the economy (and to this extent we consider the crisis as having as exogenous source), while other

DOI: 10.4324/9781003153900-4

economic downturns used as benchmarks against which the pandemic crisis is compared emerged from within the economy (and, therefore, they are considered as having an endogenous source) (Delatte and Guillaume, 2020). This, in itself, shows the differences between the economic consequences of the pandemic crisis and previous economic crises. The sense of emergency and the awareness of the potential devastating effects of the pandemic crisis (here envisaged at the economic level only) asked for massive government intervention. A vast array of public subsidies aimed at preventing the destruction of the economy and massive disbursements on national healthcare systems that met the sanitary challenges of the crisis justified an abrupt and overwhelming deterioration of fiscal deficits and the public debt–GDP ratio. Suddenly, contingency legitimised a U-turn on the mainstream political-economic rationale concerning fiscal policy. This was not the time for governments to comply with fiscal discipline. From fiscal surpluses or small fiscal deficits, countries suddenly turned into substantial fiscal deficits and worsened public indebtedness.

Section 3.4 focuses on the EU's economic policy response to the pandemic crisis. With the ghost of the Eurozone crisis still lingering, sudden economic challenges stemming from the quick spread of the disease surfaced. EU institutions were able to agree on special mechanisms to stifle the negative impact of the pandemic on member states' economies. The reaction was much quicker than in the case of the Eurozone crisis, although EU institutions did not supply their input at the same time.

Finally, Section 3.5 places the analysis within the normative dimension. Important lessons are to be drawn from the economic policy designed to prevent the collapse of economic activity and from the necessary adjustment to the economic effects of the sanitary crisis. To what extent is the economic policy shift consistent with an adjusted rationale, one that is inconsistent with the prevailing political-economic paradigm? Discussion takes place at two different levels. On the one hand, by asking whether a different economic policy template emerged from political-economic reactions to the pandemic crisis. Discussion revolves around whether emergency economic policy is typical of a political-economic rationale different from the one that prevailed before the crisis emerged. On the other hand, discussion addresses how congruent is it to consider an economic policy shift considering that the times in which such shift happened were (are) exceptional. In other words, to what extent exceptional measures qualify to recognise a new political-economic paradigm following governments' (also the European Union's) reactions to the pandemic crisis?

3.2 The impact on GDP, inflation and unemployment

Immediate challenges of the sanitary crisis were visible in the form of a sudden drop of economic activity (Fernandes, 2020). Faced with a highly contagious disease, governments had to resort to an overarching lockdown. The emergency and ensuing governments' panic coupled with the scientific community

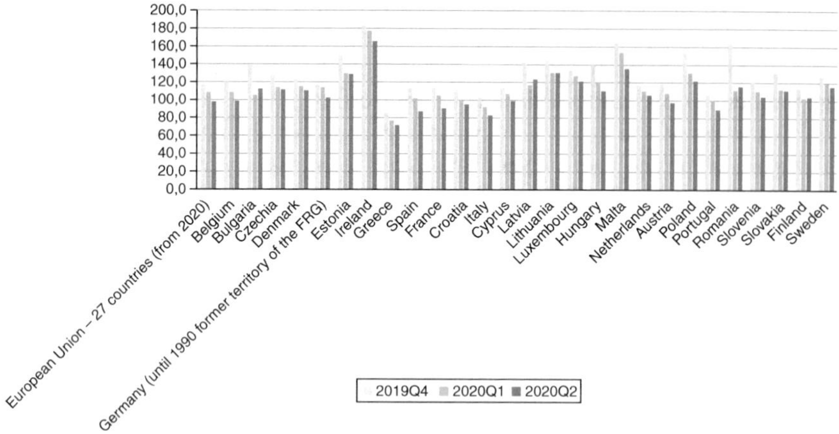

Figure 3.1 GDP evolution, 2019–2020, member states of the European Union.

Source: Eurostat (2020). *GDP and Main Components (Output, Expenditure and Income), Gross Domestic Product at Market Prices*. Available at: https://ec.europa.eu/eurostat/web/national-accounts/data/main-tables [Accessed 2 December 2020].

haphazard learning process of the COVID-19 virus forced authorities to implement radical measures. The propagation of the virus had to be tamed somehow. Stopping many economic activities was among the urgent decisions implemented by national authorities.

Lockdown represented a huge setback to many economic sectors. Services at large were heavily impacted. Hotels, restaurants and companies producing non-fundamental commodities had to stop functioning (Gourinchas, Kalemli-Özcan, Penciakova and Sander, 2020). This represented an immense drop on production and consumption, with a catastrophic effect on GDP and unemployment. Since the economy went to a standstill, governments became aware that urgent solutions were required to stop the economy from massive stumbling down. Temporary measures aiming at preserving workers' earnings were necessary. Otherwise, economic downfall would have been more severe, for the marked impact on unemployment. The chain of events that interlaces consumption and production could trigger a severe economic depression.

Amidst bewilderment at the outset of COVID-19 outbreak, governments' utmost goal was the mitigation of negative consequences. At some point, a trade-off between lockdown and the preservation of economic activity was at stake, especially after political authorities realised the massive impact on the economy after they decided to enforce lockdown (Goolsbee and Syverson, 2020). The deterioration of GDP and unemployment figures shocked decision-makers. According to statistical data (see Figures 3.1 and 3.2), the fall on GDP was unprecedented.

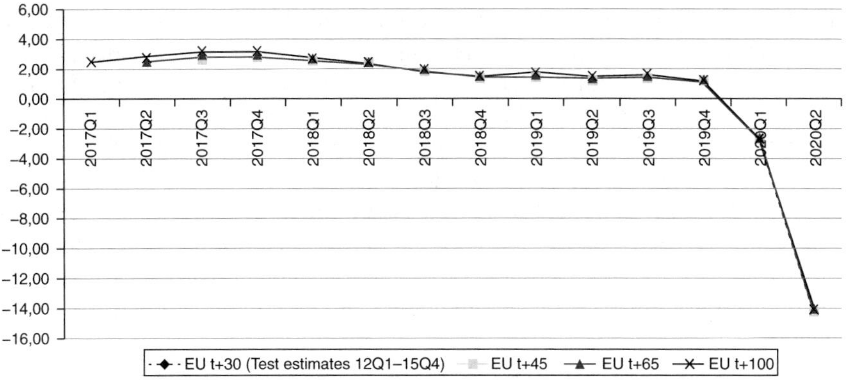

Figure 3.2 GDP evolution, 2019–2020, European Union.

Source: Eurostat (2020). *EU GDP Aggregate Revision Triangles*. Available at: https://ec.europa.eu/eurostat/web/national-accounts/data/other [Accessed 2 December 2020].

Data show how the economic implications of COVID-19 pandemic puts the EU economy at the edge of a dramatic economic crisis. At the end of the second quarter of 2020, GDP dropped to −14 per cent. Observers might be attracted to engage on a comparison with the Great Depression of the 1930s in order to find out similarities and differences between both episodes of crisis (Susskind and Vines, 2020). This is, nonetheless, a flawed exercise. On the one hand, the underlying reasons for both crises are different. While the depression of the 1930s was caused by economic factors only, the ongoing crisis was fed by an exogenous source. A sanitary crisis with assorted ramifications had detrimental effects on the economy. The uniqueness of the sanitary crisis (notably the characteristics of the virus) triggered a sudden and deep impact on the economy. On the other hand, despite contagious effects of the depression of the 1930s enabling a quick externalisation of the crisis, on the current crisis negative spillovers acted much quickly as the channels of contamination (the disease and its economic consequences) have a dimension that makes comparisons with the 1930s meaningless (Sachs, 2020).

The same line of reasoning rules out the comparison between the pandemic crisis and the Eurozone crisis. While the Eurozone crisis was an asymmetric crisis (the sovereign debt crisis hit a few member states) (Giavazzi and Wyplosz, 2015), economic implications of the pandemic crisis have a symmetric nature (Tesche, 2020). Figures on the evolution of the GDP are the instructive evidence. One way or another, all EU member states were severely affected, notwithstanding differences emerge from a cross-country analysis. Yet, and importantly, no EU member state escaped to the devastating effects on economic growth.

The consequences on economic growth were disturbing. Economic activity suddenly dropped when citizens had to stay at home for a period of time. The economy did not fully stop, as basic supplies were still being produced, notably foodstuff. The retail sector was also functioning, as people needed to buy basic commodities for their daily survival. Other than that, the economy was brought to a halt. Figures concerning GDP are therefore not surprising. This, in turn, posed governments a new challenge. They had to design measures to absorb the negative implications of the economic crisis. Additional challenges to fiscal policy were at stake, as governments had to plan emergency measures aiming at some preservation of citizens' income and companies' earnings (see Section 3.3 for the analysis of the impact of the pandemic crisis on public finances).

Despite lockdown affecting many economic activities, the negative impact on unemployment was toned-down by emergency measures implemented by governments. Workers were reassured to some extent. Many jobs were lost (Gallant, Kroft, Lange and Notowidigdo, 2020). In other cases, temporary measures were designed to protect jobs and to maintain – as much as possible – workers' income. Layoff programmes became generalised (Wolcott, Ochse, Kudlyak and Kouchekinia, 2020). This exceptional measure protected the job market from devastating effects. Layoff saved many jobs. On the one hand, it implied a cost for the government, as financial compensation owing to layoff measures required massive payments. On the other hand, layoff also added a financial burden to companies themselves, as the typical design of layoff measures involved co-responsibility between the government and companies (Bartik et al., 2020). Companies faced a decrease of production that heavily impacted on their revenue and, on the top of this, they were asked to partially ensure layoff compensation payments. A double-edged sword hit many companies. Lower production implied a decrease of income. Nevertheless, companies were asked to pay an amount of layoff payments. This added to many companies' fragile financial situation.

Losses on the job market were not so sharp as the drop of GDP implies, as data on Figure 3.3 show.

A comparison of data on Figures 3.1 and 3.2, on the one hand, and Figure 3.3 shows how different the impact was. The decrease of economic activity was deeper than the negative consequences on the job market. Despite correlation exists between both variables, the testable hypothesis is whether emergency measures aiming at protecting workers' income explain the gap between the losses on economic growth and the increase on unemployment. Yet, losses on the labour market were considerable, as the comparison between unemployment rates in 2019 and 2020 reveals. In addition, the domestic impact of jobs' losses was far from being evenly distributed across the society, as there is evidence that fragile groups of the labour market (youngsters, part-time jobs, workers with a fragile labour market position) were more affected than groups enjoying a stable position (Fana, Torrejón Pérez and Fernández-Macías, 2020). One of the negative consequences of the economic dimension

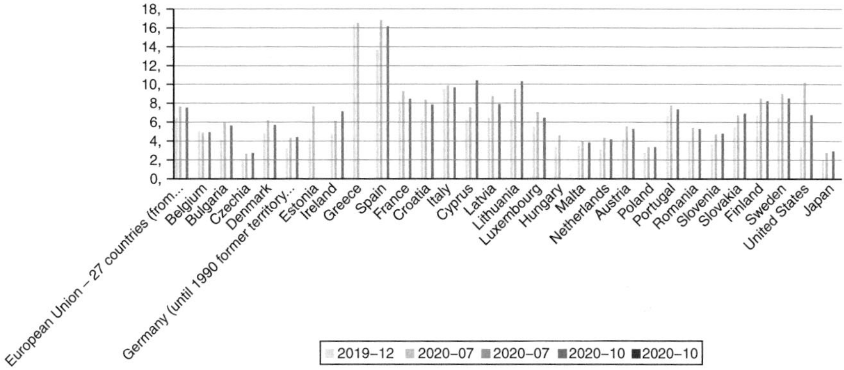

Figure 3.3 Evolution of unemployment, 2019–2020, member states of the EU.

Source: Eurostat (2020). *Harmonised Unemployment Rate by Sex*. Available at: https://ec.europa.eu/eurostat/en/web/products-datasets/-/TEILM020 [Accessed 3 December 2020].

of the pandemic crisis was the widening of differences between unprotected workers and those who benefit from higher protection standards.

Negative effects on the labour market also heightened economic downfall. A drop on production lowers consumption, as companies severely hit had to close doors and make a considerable number of workers unemployed. Despite providing unemployed persons with subsidies, the pattern over time shows a decrease in consumption as unemployed workers suffering a loss of income (the unemployment subsidy does not match previous earnings) reacted cautiously, anticipating a potential long-term cut in income if they stay outside the labour market for a long period. At the same time, cuts on workers' earnings (those who were laid-off) lead to decreased consumption and had an impact on production at a later stage. In addition to the first wave of production and consumption losses triggered by the direct impact of the political economy of the COVID-19 pandemic, a second wave was observed. The underlying reasons come from the consequences of the pandemic on the economy. The second wave, in turn, further depressed the economy.

The combination of these factors also impacted on inflation. Data on Figure 3.4 address the evolution of inflation on a cross-country, intertemporal analysis.

The major explanation for lower inflation is connected with the economic turmoil that came after the economy was hit by the sanitary crisis. The deterioration of consumption and production explains, to a large extent, why inflation decelerated and came into figures consistent with deflation in many countries (Denmark, Estonia, Ireland, Greece, Spain, Croatia, Cyprus, Latvia, Luxembourg, Portugal, Slovenia, Finland and Sweden). Interestingly,

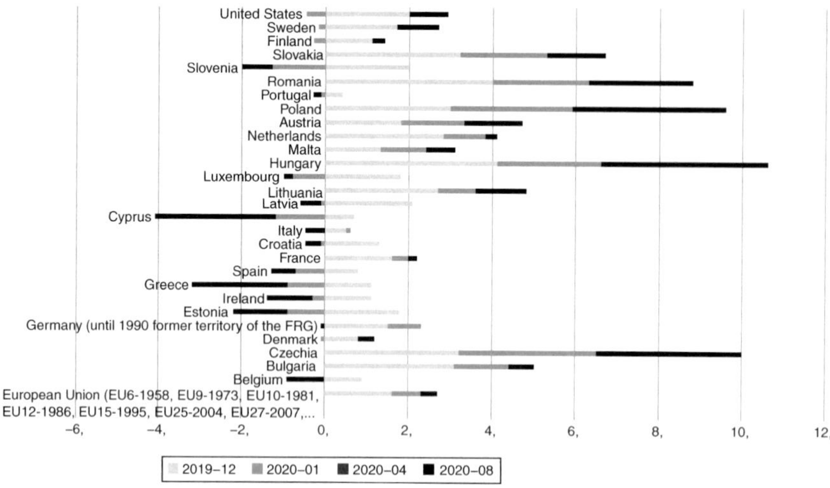

Figure 3.4 Evolution of inflation, 2019–2020, member states of the EU.

Source: Eurostat (2020). *HICP (2015=100) – monthly data (annual rate of change)*. Available at: https://ec.europa.eu/eurostat/web/covid-19/data [Accessed 3 December 2020].

not only these countries are not a majority of member states but crucially the largest economies were able to escape deflation. Production cuts, especially the drop in consumption, added further strain on the markets. Lockdown also added psychological effects that impacted on consumers' behaviour (Sheth, 2020). Faced with the unprecedented slowdown of economic activity and fearing that they could be next to be affected by a loss of income, demand suffered considerable cuts and exposed supply to additional factors of stress. Overall, this pattern is consistent with a demand shock that pushed prices downwards (Barrero, Bloom and Davis, 2020).

Perhaps this effect is surprising (if the psychological reaction of consumers is not encompassed), since extraordinary government measures designed to protect workers' earnings were theoretically expected to mitigate the decrease of consumption. While consumption obviously dampened the economic sectors subjected to a total lockdown, other economic activities did not suffer. While consumers were not affected on the provision of fundamental commodities, the economy at large was considerably affected by the lockdown. If scholars who argue that consumers are risk-averse have a point, this might be an explanation for the rapid and sharp decrease of consumption with side-effects on the evolution of inflation (Carlsson-Szlezak, Reeves and Swartz, 2020). The crucial aspect to be included in the analysis is the awareness of uncertainty regarding the evolution of the pandemics and to what extent more severe effects on the economy were to be expected (McKibbin and Roshen, 2020).

Surprisingly, for a sudden and deep loss of GDP a sharper decrease of inflation was to be expected, as the breakdown of economic activity feeds a deflationary process (Ilzetzki, Reinhart and Rogoff, 2020). Regardless of the devastating impact on the economy (as measured by the evolution of GDP), inflation fared relatively well, as data on Figure 3.4 confirm. The steeper curve regarding the evolution of GDP shows how moderate the contagious effect to inflation was. According to the literature (Jaravel and O'Connell, 2020), unprecedented losses on GDP, and the speed that these losses contaminated the economy with, explain why the impact on inflation was less marked.

3.3 The impact on public finances

When countries are knocked by an economic crisis, public finances deteriorate. Mainstream understanding is that automatic stabilisers operate in order to smooth the negative effects of the economic crisis (Paulus and Tasseva, 2020). If unemployment rises, social security payments will increase, since unemployed persons are entitled to receive a subsidy that compensates them for staying outside the labour market. Together with other negative effects on fiscal policy on government's budget income (with depressed economic activity, tax collection drops), growing public deficit is correlated with a negative business cycle.

Considering the devastating effects of the pandemic crisis on GDP (as the previous section documented), it was expected that member states' fiscal policies would also be affected. The sudden deterioration of economic activity had an impact on the collection of several categories of taxes and on public spending (Casado et al., 2020):

i Decreased production was the underlying reason of companies' losses, which, in turn, determined a decrease on the collection of companies' profit tax.

ii Cuts on production also triggered diminishing consumption (which, in turn, was heightened not only by the effects of lockdown, but also because many persons' earnings decreased). The collection of the consumption tax (value added tax) dropped accordingly.

iii Faced with lower production, companies fired workers. Their wage disbursement was therefore lower. This, in turn, fed a decrease on governments' collection of taxes on wages.

iv Governments supported jobless persons, therefore increasing the amount of unemployment subsidies. This was one the sources of the increase on public spending.

v In addition, all emergency measures to mitigate the deceleration of economic activity, notably payments regarding layoff measures, represented a burden for governments.

vi Finally, public spending also increased due to the needs of national healthcare systems (more funds made available to hospitals when they were faced with a massive demand of infected persons and the broadening of detection tests).

Statistical data confirm crowding out effects of the pandemic crisis on public finances. An introductory remark is necessary though: the effects on fiscal policy were, in turn, the consequence of the impact of the pandemic crisis on economic activity. What is implied is the recognition of cascading effects: the pandemic was the reason why the economy suffered so much; the consequence of economic deceleration was the deterioration of public finances in all the EU member states.

As far as the fiscal deficit is concerned, data on Figure 3.5 show how deep the deterioration was. Sound fiscal policy (which, in turn, was made possible by the favourable economic outlook of the previous five years) (De Grauwe and Ji, 2019) was suddenly replaced by high fiscal deficits and prospects for an increase on the public debt/GDP ratio (see Figure 3.6). All of a sudden, member states would fall into positions consistent with unsound fiscal policy, wasn't for the exceptional macroeconomic conditions that justified the suspension of the Eurozone's fiscal rules (the Stability and Growth Pact and the Fiscal Pact) (Constantini, 2020). The combination of opposing effects – cuts on public revenue and exacerbated public spending – was amplified by the dimension of the economic crisis.

Worsened fiscal policy positions were innate to the new macroeconomic conditions triggered by the pandemic crisis. Yet, at the same time, concerns emerged about the sudden and harsh deterioration of the fiscal deficit and the prospects for a considerable increase of public indebtedness. On the one hand, memories of the Eurozone crisis were still vivid, albeit observers and decision-makers were consensual in pointing out the differences between the pandemic crisis and the Eurozone crisis (Borio, 2020). On the other hand, the awareness of government intervention to meet the economic challenges

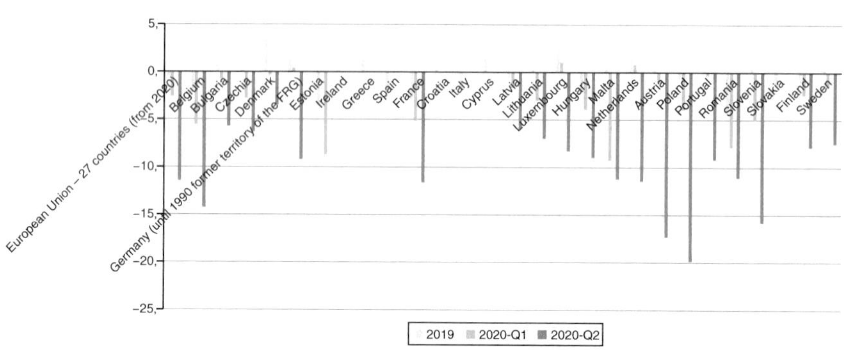

Figure 3.5 Evolution of the public deficit (2019–2020), member states of the EU.

Source: Eurostat (2020). *General government deficit/surplus*. Available at: https://ec.europa.eu/eurostat/web/covid-19/data [Accessed 3 December 2020].

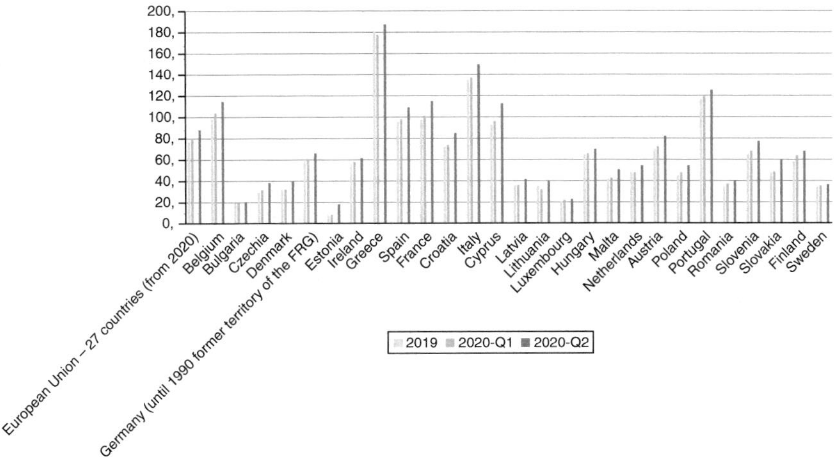

Figure 3.6 Evolution of public debt/GDP (2019–2020, estimations), member states of the EU.

Source: Eurostat (2020). *General government gross debt*. Available at: https://ec.europa.eu/eurostat/web/covid-19/data [Accessed 3 December 2020].

stemming from the pandemic crisis threw into the air an additional reason of concern. First, governments needed resources to validate their reaction to the sudden economic crisis that soon hit countries. Higher fiscal deficits and, especially, the negative outlook for the medium-term evolution of public debt could nurture restrictions on governments' capacity to provide an appropriate answer. In addition, the severe impact on fiscal policy could also derail countries' positions in the future, extending the temporal dimension of the crisis because of medium- to long-term implications of the crisis on fiscal policy.

Governments were pressured by a paradox. Private economic agents were anaemic, which explains why economic activity almost stopped. To prevent mounting pressures of the crisis from taking place, governments' intervention was required and urgent (Benmelehc and Tzur-Ilan, 2020). The first wave of governments' interventions was one justification of the severe impact on fiscal policy (the other being the natural decrease on budget revenue that came from tax collection, for the reasons mentioned above). Governments could not refrain from supporting the economy, which heightened the fiscal deficit and added extra pressure on member states' public debt sustainability. The explosive combination of rising public indebtedness with decreasing GDP deteriorated the public debt/GDP ratio.

Rising public debt could spread mistrust among markets. Looking back at the sovereign debt crisis, a sort of self-fulfilling prophecy acted against the sustainability of some member states' public debt, as rising public debt/GDP ratio pushed market agents to put a higher risk premium on these countries' public debt (Mody, 2018). This, in turn, amplified the difficulties surrounding the management of public debt, as higher interest rates increased the burden of the public debt. Consequently, the debt/GDP ratio boosted further as a result of a twofold, coincident process: the rise on interest rates also raised the stock of public debt, but it also deteriorated the ratio vis-à-vis GDP as the countries mostly affected were still suffering from negative economic growth. Despite lessons from the Eurozone crisis were still fresh, markets were aware that this time the source of the economic crisis that impacted on member states' fiscal policy was different (Li, Strahan and Zhang, 2020). It was not an outcome of wrong policy choices adding to the pile of public debt (as markets perceived the Eurozone crisis at that time).[1]

The economic dimension of the crisis was a side-effect of an overarching crisis that was, first and foremost, sanitary. Notwithstanding markets' perception of the different nature of the current crisis and the Eurozone crisis, it was feared that mounting pressures on public debt sustainability could emerge if and when massive public deficits prompted a sizeable deterioration of the public debt/GDP ratio. Governments needed leverage to implement the new archetype of economic policy required by the exceptional circumstances of the pandemic crisis. Massive interventionism was not consistent with prudential fiscal policy, as it is commensurate when markets (i.e., creditors) assess countries' reputation as debtors.

Hence, after the first weeks of national authorities' bewilderment on how to cope with the pandemic crisis, finally governments realised that a coordinated, EU-wide answer was required for the terrific consequences of the pandemic and the challenges for the economy. EU institutions were the appropriate locus for the reaction of political authorities to the economic dimension of the pandemic crisis. This time, the EU did not lag behind the challenges of the crisis and reacted promptly.

3.4 The economic policy reaction of the European Union

At the outset, national governments' narrow-minded approach neglected cooperation. Soon after coronavirus socked Europe, the contagious effects of the pandemic crisis and the anticipated devastating social and economic consequences were acknowledged by national authorities. They decided to articulate within the European Council. The ECB and the Commission acted on their own, with disparate degrees of influence.

The role of the ECB during the Eurozone crisis is useful to assess the central bank's approach to COVID-19. Unlike the early stages of the Eurozone crisis, the ECB was not trapped on inertia when economic turmoil emerged. The ECB was swift to anticipate the negative effects of the economic crisis (Giavazzi and Tabellini, 2020). The Outright Monetary Transactions (OMT) programme was the standpoint for the ECB's action. On 18 March 2020 a new vehicle, the PEPP, paved the way for the ECB to buy up to €750 billion of member states' public debt on the secondary market (Lucchese and Pianta, 2020). Member states were given room of manoeuvre to resort to fiscal policy.

The ECB reacted quickly, taking a proactive approach. The central bank anticipated the macroeconomic symptoms of the crisis, creating a financial vehicle to address future challenges. The ECB's position was strengthened on 4 June 2020 when the Governing Council decided to almost double the PEPP capacity up to €1,350 trillion (European Central Bank, 2020a). Since forecasts of the economic impact of the pandemic crisis were reviewed (pushing the negative effects upwards), the ECB decided to reinforce the protective belt against the destructive effects of the pandemic crisis. The monetary authority decided to further increase the PEPP capacity with an additional €500 billion on the 10 December 2020 meeting of the Governing Council, expanding the duration of the programme until March 2022. The ECB is expected to buy up to €1,850 trillion of member states' public debt (European Central Bank, 2020b).

At the same time, the ECB asked national governments to resort to fiscal activism. It was a paradigm shift in the Eurozone governance. In the past, the ECB frequently constrained national governments' latitude on fiscal policy, considering fiscal discipline a key aspect of EMU. Faced with the challenges of the pandemic crisis, the ECB changed its approach. The central bank recognised the important role of fiscal policy in order to overcome the economic crisis. Before the outbreak of the sanitary crisis, the ECB pointed out that the expansion of countries' public spending was crucial to accelerate economic activity and to enable economic growth.[2] Since fighting the economic crisis was the priority for economic policymaking, the appeal of the ECB was rational.

OMT and PEPP give ground to national governments' resort to fiscal activism. Although the ECB created the conditions for fiscal activism, national governments have to play their role. This is why the ECB has been asking national governments for a firm commitment to increasing public spending as the appropriate fiscal stimulus in times of economic crisis. ECB's intervention on public debt's secondary market is far from being enough. The central bank seeks national governments' co-responsibility for economic recovery, thus lessening the risk of moral hazard, which puts the 'frugal four' (Netherlands, Denmark, Austria and Finland) and the 'cohesion countries' against each other. Fiscal activism upgrades national governments' standard of responsibility. Thus, the ECB acted as a decisive, although discrete, leader in the context of the Eurozone's macroeconomic adjustment to the sanitary crisis.

The European Council failed to take the centre stage, at least at the initial stages of the crisis. The institution did not react so quickly as the ECB or the Commission. Since national authorities have a seat in the European Council, it is understandable that inertia upsets decision-making. For more sensitive decisions, consensus is required. When national interests clash, decision-making becomes prone to veto points and it is the outcome of a cumbersome process. Decisions are often postponed until veto players are convinced and give their agreement (Frieden and Walter, 2019).

At the beginning, discussions focused on how to support national economies. The strengthening of EMU was at stake in early discussions, since the strong likelihood of economic disruption with asymmetric effects triggered new challenges. In the event of overwhelming macroeconomic forecasts, issues such as risk-sharing and Eurobonds (renamed Coronabonds) reappeared (Herzog, 2020). These discussions started in the academia and the press. Nevertheless, the discussion reached the political level. The European Council could not avoid the discussion. Debates were aggressive and hostile, as different stances were voiced with vehemence and animosity. Unable to reach an agreement on the details of a common solution, the European Council eventually instructed the Commission to design a recovery plan. Hesitation aired in the European Council's meetings, and a unanimous agreement was not possible. Arguably, by asking the Commission to prepare a detailed proposal for the near future, the European Council bought some time.

Meanwhile, important events disturbed the timeline of the pandemic crisis in the EU. On the 5 May 2020, the German Constitutional Court challenged the European Court of Justice's (ECJ) ruling that endorsed the legal background of the OMT programme (BVerfG, 2020). The German Constitutional Court defied the ECB to provide legal arguments within three months. The timing of the German Constitutional Court was not innocent. The ECB had just announced the PEPP to accommodate the expected effects of the economic crisis. Some days later (18 May 2020), the German chancellor Angela Merkel and the French president Emmanuel Macron announced a joint plan for the recovery of the EU of the pandemic crisis.[3] Both countries were politically willing to create a massive recovery plan made partially of grants and partially of loans. A Franco-German initiative triggered the initiative in the EU, as it happened many times in the past. This time Germany did not resist to a more ambitious solution that involved higher disbursements and a burden to German taxpayers. It remains to be seen whether this initiative was the political reaction to the drama activated by the constitutional doubts of the German Constitutional Court.

Germany and France joint action gave moral authority to the Commission's soon-to-be recovery plan. However, well before issuing its recovery plan, the Commission's activism in responding to the different dimensions of the crisis (see Chapter 2), including the economic dimension, was manifest. For example, on 10 March 2020, the Commission's President announced a Corona Response Investment Initiative (CRII) with a €37 billion envelope under the cohesion policy, while proposing measures to ease the negative impact of the COVID-19 outbreak on the aviation industry and the environment. The CRII was submitted three days later. The Commission's proposals included:

i arranging EU budget instruments to immediately alleviate firms, sectors of activity and regions seriously affected by the pandemic;

ii state aid delivered to citizens and national companies, authorising full flexibility within state aid rules to support the economy battered by COVID-19;
iii boosting banking sector liquidity, enlarging the scope of the Solidarity Fund to include major public health crises; and
iv flexibility of Eurozone's fiscal rules through the activation of the general escape clause of the Stability and Growth Pact to accommodate fiscal activism (European Commission, 2020).

Commission's proposals were endorsed by the Eurogroup and the European Council (Eurogroup, 2020; European Council/Council of the European Union, 2020a). Commission's activism peaked, with proposals and measures submitted on a regular basis. The SURE[4] initiative (2 April), adopted by the Council on 19 May 2020, a solidarity instrument supporting member states' initiatives to protect employment, is just an example. Internal measures were paired with a continuous effort to put together a global response to the pandemic, namely by securing financial support to partner countries through EU external action funds and programmes. The Commission also implemented several initiatives to raise funds to help financing the fight against coronavirus around the world, of which the *Global Goal: Unite for Our Future* pledging summit is just an example. Also, the Commission joined the COVID-19 Vaccine Global Access Facility (known as COVAX), a global risk-sharing mechanism for pooled procurement and equitable access to affordable COVID-19 vaccines.

As the economic dimension of the crisis emancipated from the health dimension (the numbers of COVID-19 infections increased and devastating economic forecasts emerged), the need to design a robust recovery plan similar the one that lifted Europe's economy after World War II became extremely pressing. Many voices pleaded for a second Marshal Plan. Following the 26 March 2020 European Council's request (European Council/Council of the European Union, 2020c), the presidents of the Commission and of the European Council presented a *Joint European Roadmap towards Lifting COVID-19 Containment Measures* (15 April 2020), aiming at bringing Europe's societies and economies back to a normal functioning as well as to prepare the ground for a comprehensive recovery plan. In the 23 April 2020 meeting, the European Council charged the Commission to submit a proposal on a buffer to the economic effects of the crisis (European Council/Council of the European Union, 2020b). Despite the urgency of the request, it took the Commission more than one month to present the proposal (the European Commission presented the European Recovery Plan on 27 May 2020).[5] One explanation is the depth of the task endorsed to the Commission. The design of an ambitious plan to boost the EU's economy that at the same time overcame member states' differences on the size or the type of instruments to channel the funds (e.g., grants or loans) was a difficult endeavour.

The Plan foresees a €750 billion European Recovery Instrument (dubbed Next Generation EU). The Commission, on behalf of the EU, will borrow on the financial markets €750 billion for the recovery fund. These funds will be repaid through future EU budgets (from 2028 to 2058). In addition, the Commission presented a revamped proposal for the next MFF (amounting to €1,100 billion between 2021 and 2027) and an updated Commission work programme for 2020 (European Commission, 2020, p. 4). The money raised through Next Generation EU (€500 billion in grants and €250 billion in loans) and the new EU budget will be delivered through EU programmes and invested across three pillars (European Commission, 2020, pp. 4–6):

i support member states' investment and reforms, including a new "Recovery and Resilience Facility" totalling €560 billion (of which €310 billion in grants and €250 billion in loans) to help member states in funding recovery and resilience plans, and a new initiative REACT-EU (Recovery Assistance for Cohesion and the Territories of Europe) for crisis repair measures;
ii reanimating the EU economy by providing incentives to private investment, which includes upgrading InvestEU and creating a Strategic Investment Facility and a new Solvency Support Instrument;
iii a new standalone EU4Health Programme for prevention and crisis preparedness and to boost the support to EU global partners through the enhancement of existing external cooperation and aid instruments.

The plan was first addressed on the 19 June European Council meeting, where disagreements were noticed. The decision of the European Council came on mid-July 2020, when the institution finally met on a face-to-face format, almost five months after the outbreak of the pandemic crisis and the recognition of the soon-to-come economic crisis.

The majority of member states welcomed the Commission's proposal[6] and considered it a good 'starting point'. However, the 'frugal four'[7] opposed to debt mutualisation and to the increase of the EU budget. The Commission's methodology for channelling funds to member states was contested by several countries (Netherlands, Denmark, Austria, Belgium, Ireland, Lithuania and Hungry) for having no connection with the pandemic, anticipating the complexity of the negotiations ahead. Nonetheless, the urgency of the response prevailed. The recovering package went through an unusually fast legislative procedure. After reaching a preliminary agreement in November 2020, the Council and the EP negotiators reached a political agreement in December on the Recovery and Resilience Facility, the key programme at the heart of Next Generation EU.

The EP approved the Facility on 9 February 2021 and the Council adopted it on 11 February 2021. The final act was published in the Official Journal of the EU on 18 February 2021 and came into force the following day. In order to benefit from the facility, member states had to prepare recovery and resilience national plans (the plans were expected to be formally submitted by 30 April 2021) setting out a package of reforms and public investment projects (to be implemented by 2026). Each plan was expected to contribute to the four dimensions outlined in the 2021 Annual Sustainable Growth Strategy (environmental sustainability, productivity, fairness, macroeconomic stability).

These plans will be assessed by the Commission and approved by the Council. The agreement between the Council and the EP on the REACT-EU was reached at interinstitutional negotiations (trilogue) on 18 November 2020. The REACT-EU Regulation came into force on 24 December 2020. Also on December 2020, after receiving the EP's consent, the Council unanimously adopted the Regulation laying down the EU's MFF for the 2021–27 period. As for the EU4Health Programme, the EP and the Council reached an agreement in March 2021.

3.5 The political economy of the pandemic crisis: is there a place for a normative assessment?

Apparently, the exceptional circumstances of the pandemic crisis were fertile ground for a paradigm shift on economic policymaking. The unprecedented crisis that stumbled over the economy required a different approach on two co-related areas. First, the sudden drop of economic activity raised unique challenges for policymakers. Emergency economic policy should tackle the corrosive effects of a massive downfall. Second, after a few weeks of hesitation, national governments finally realised that joint action was essential to mitigate the immediate negative economic effects tied to the sanitary crisis. EU institutions took centre stage again. With the benefit of hindsight, lessons from the recent Eurozone crisis were captured. Not that the pandemic crisis is comparable to the Eurozone crisis. EU institutions were not expected to fall into the trap of inertia, as they did for an extended period before action was undertaken after some member states were beleaguered with public debt unsustainability. This time was to be different, as the prospect of a deep economic crisis with no feasible forecast of recovery daunted politicians in EU institutions and national governments. Protracted reaction would only exacerbate problems already affecting national economies. EU institutions were expected to shift from slow reaction stance towards proactive stance.

From the point of view of economics, an interesting discussion is whether the preconditions for a paradigm shift on economic policymaking encompass a normative dimension attached. In a monetary union largely influenced by ordo-liberalism and the monetarist school did challenges stemming from economic policy adjustment to the consequences of the pandemic crisis throw the seeds of paradigm shift, this time at the level of economics per se? Indeed, the perception on how economic policy adjustment should take place was consensual. Faced with the breakdown of many economic activities and ensuing difficulties, with a paralysis of private economic agents, all eyes turned into government action (Eichenbaum, Rebelo and Trabandt, 2020).

A revival of Keynesian-style economic policy was inexorable, indeed the only solution designed to sustain the devastating effects of economic collapse from taking place (short-term goal of economic policy) and to promote the conditions of economic recovery (medium-term goal of economic policy). The revival of Keynesianism was not an originality in the recent past. During the economic crisis, and especially in 2009, national governments resorted to a Keynesian-led economic policy aiming at lifting the economy from a sudden and deep crisis right after the world economy was affected by the financial crisis that started in the United States (Mitchell, 2015). The return to Keynesianism was short-lived, though. At that time, many economists asserted that 'we are all Keynesians now' (Stiglitz, 2013). The sentence echoed again when the economy witnessed the first signs of a deep recession right after the sanitary crisis spread to Europe (and elsewhere).

To this extent, does it make sense to bring a normative dimension into the analysis of the economic aspects of the pandemic crisis? Apparently, it does. The persuasion of many observers' accounts on the demise of the monetarist school (and of neoliberalism) seems to point at this direction. 'We are all Keynesians', again (Velasco, 2020). The new roadmap of economic policy seems consistent with the Keynesian paradigm. This, in turn, is envisaged as the withdrawal of the monetarist, ordo-liberal template of economic policy-making that influenced EMU from scratch. The focus on government intervention is characteristic of the Keynesian school. Also, the awareness that the appropriate combination of fiscal and monetary policy puts the emphasis on the former is an additional evidence of a new paradigm of economic policy. Adding to this perception, the ECB has been putting pressure on national governments to increase public investment in order to promote robust economic growth on national economies generally characterised by anaemic economic growth. If the central bank itself acknowledges the role of fiscal policy, does this tantamount to a regime shift in EMU?

To start with, the normative analysis is still provisional, as the second and the third waves of COVID-19 (at the time of writing: early April 2021) brought the prospect of a W-shaped economic recovery (Barbieri Góes and Gallo, 2020), and not a V-shaped, as several economists and international organisations predicted when the first lockdown was lifted, and signs of economic recovery were consistent (Ambrocio, 2020). Conclusions beforehand are prone to precipitation, as it was abundantly clear with categorical judgements that 'we (were) all Keynesians now'. Although the evidence so far seems to confirm the conversion of economic policy to a Keynesian-led model, additional aspects must be considered in order to temper the conclusion.

To start with, economic policy adjustment is typical of the Keynesian school. However, the rift between the two major schools of economic thought became blurred with time, as both underwent evolution (Clift, 2020). Yet, basic characteristics of the monetarist and the Keynesian schools show how contrasting they are on several areas of economic policy (Kindleberger, 2006).

Monetarists are prone to choose long-term price stability as the macroeconomic priority, while Keynesians are more sensitive to job creation and the promotion of economic growth. The monetarist design of economic policy is geared towards the medium to long term. Keynesians look after short-term necessities that influence the accommodation of economic policy. The monetarist school choses a combination of economic policy instruments that puts the emphasis on monetary policy, leaving fiscal policy to play a secondary role. Keynesians focus on fiscal policy and put monetary policy at the service of the fiscal policy agenda.

Viewed from this perspective, economic policy designed to mitigate the implications of the economic crisis seems to be in line with the Keynesian school (Skidelsky, 2020). Not only inflation is not a problem (as it wasn't prior to the pandemic crisis, it must be noted), but also contingency throws emergency into the table, which is instructive of an economic policy shaped in the short term. In addition, the recognition that government intervention is required to address the negative business cycle connected with the sanitary crisis shifts the emphasis from monetary policy to fiscal policy. Indeed, one of the first decisions of the Commission was to suspend fiscal rules that impose fiscal discipline on the Eurozone's member states (see Section 3.4). To this extent, evidence is consistent with a paradigm shift showing how economic policy accommodated to the economic challenges of the pandemic crisis, facilitating the rehabilitation of Keynesian-led economic policy.

Secondly, economists influenced by the monetarist school recognised that there is room for fiscal policy and government interventionism when the economy is severely affected by a crisis of the kind of the current one (Modigliani, 1977). As mentioned before, not only the divide between the two schools of economic thought is not a matter of strict binary analysis, but the lines of dissention between them are prone to flexibility when special circumstances underline the business cycle. Monetarists not only do not neglect a role for fiscal policy under normal circumstances, but they acknowledge that when a severe crisis hits the economy fiscal activism ranks high in the appropriate economic policy mix.

For example, when the Stability and Growth Pact (SGP) was added to the rules that govern EMU, a discussion between the critics and those who accepted the SGP took place. Critics argued that the SGP constrained national authorities' fiscal policy, as they estimated that the Eurozone's fiscal rule intensified the bias in favour of monetary policy and further limited the leeway of fiscal policy (Heipertz and Verdun, 2010). Those who argued in favour of the SGP had a different rationale. Since the SGP imposed a straitjacket on member states' fiscal deficit (GDP 3 per cent) and advised to bring it closer to zero or in surplus, it was argued that fiscal policy should closely follow the needs of the business cycle. National governments ought to seize the opportunity of booms to bring the fiscal deficit close to zero or in surplus so that when a crisis plunged the economy automatic stabilisers would operate, allowing the fiscal deficit to naturally go up (Artis and Buti, 2000). The rationale of automatic stabilisers is purported by the Keynesian school, not so much by monetarists (Eichengreen, 2020).

Thirdly, the argument that the ECB opened the window of opportunity to fiscal activism and, hence, to government intervention deserves qualification. Before the outbreak of COVID-19, the central bank already claimed that national governments should increase public investment so that they would provide their input to robust economic growth. The position of the ECB is to be understood within the proper context, which leads the reader to remember that the decisions and actions of the central bank were crucial to take the Eurozone away from the crisis that at some point affected fragile, peripheral, over-indebted member states (with the potential of negative externalities to other member states and to the whole Eurozone acting as a threat) (Kratochvíl and Sychra, 2019). When the ECB decided to buy public debt bonds on the secondary market, the negative trend that pushed those member states' interest rates upwards, creating serious problems of public debt unsustainability, was over. National governments could count with the ECB if economic conditions deteriorated in the future. The OMT programme set the precedent.

Faced with persistent anaemic economic growth, the ECB wanted to share responsibilities if a dauting scenario materialised. The monetary authority was ready to act accordingly. The ECB, however, did not want the full burden to fall on its shoulders. This is the rationale of the constant pledge for national governments to give their input through fiscal policy, especially after problems of over-indebtedness vanished and all countries were able to bring fiscal deficit close to zero and some of them were able to run fiscal surpluses. The ECB acted strategically, asking national governments to give their contribution with embedded co-responsibility of the actors charged of monetary and fiscal policy as the optimal solution. Such behavioural pattern of the monetary authority is not a concession to the Keynesian school whatsoever. It shows, on the other hand, how a strict analysis of conventional characteristics of both schools of economic thought is obsolete, since some of the differences that were more pronounced in the past were blurred.

Fourthly, perhaps the biggest challenge comes from the point of view of EMU's conventional template of economic policy. A cautious analysis warns how hasty conclusions are prone to be watered down. It is true that the political-economic model of EMU was accused of rigidity (Wyplosz, 2006). It is also undeniable that the Eurozone was ill-designed. This shortcoming become palpable when EMU was attacked by an asymmetric crisis that, at some point, threatened to turn into a crisis affecting the Eurozone as a whole (Fabbrini, 2013). The Eurozone was forced to adjust to the vagaries of the previous crisis and to encompass measures of reform that acknowledge how the original architecture of EMU was flawed (De Grauwe, 2015). EMU accommodated to a new context that made political institutions to recognise how the original construction should adjust to recent events, and especially how important it was to change EMU to prevent the consequences of future crises. In a nutshell, EMU showed signs of flexibility. Whether EMU policymakers were convinced of this teleological shift or their acceptance was the outcome of a strategic move is something that future historiographic accounts of these years might reveal.

3.6 Conclusions

This chapter focused on the economic dimension of the pandemic crisis. It stressed how economies were harshly affected by the economic consequences of the pandemic crisis, opening a crisis on its own (the economic crisis within the sanitary crisis). In order to fully capture the dynamics of the economic crisis, data on GDP, unemployment and inflation were assessed. Another dimension that accounted for the broad macroeconomic picture was the implications on fiscal policy. As it was expected, times of crisis raise a forceful challenge for fiscal policy. Not only the operation of automatic stabilisers puts fiscal policy under stress, but also urgent economic policy measures designed to mitigate the early effects of the crisis had a severe impact on the sustainability of public finances.

On a comparative basis, this crisis is unprecedented. Its destructive potential raised the alarm on national governments. At some point, after early misorientation and self-centredness, national authorities became aware that the fight against the economic crisis required joint action. EU institutions came to the fore. With different degrees of influence, they were able to break a long-standing tradition of inertia and gave a proactive answer to the crisis. Many of the economic policy measures approved represent a paradigm shift for European integration. To this extent, the pandemic crisis was an opportunity for change in the EU. Crucially, the economic policy reaction was swifter than in the Eurozone crisis, which is an outcome of the learning effects of the previous crisis and the recognition that with the pandemic crisis the potential for a more devastating economic and social crisis was higher.

Finally, the chapter asked whether it makes sense to embed a normative discussion to the economic policy adjustment to the pandemic crisis. Warnings about the provisional reading of measures approved are to be coupled with the undeniable changing character of economic policy and whether a paradigm shift for EMU is at stake. What remains to be seen is whether the purported political-economic regime change holds when normal times return to the cartography of EMU. The accommodation of economic policy owes to the contingency that pushed for a different economic policy mix. The proof of life of regime change (and, hence, of the normative implications of the adjustment to the economic challenges of the pandemic crisis) will come in the future. If the current economic policy mix withstands through calm waters, that will confirm how rightful it was to take a normative reading of the economic policy adjustment to the economic crisis triggered by the sanitary crisis. Otherwise, if 'business as usual' trumps, the long-standing political-economic paradigm of the Eurozone is unchanged. In that case, the hermeneutics of the current crisis as the epitome of regime change is not appropriate, as a different template of economic policy was short-lived. Time will tell.

Notes

1 Such approach to the underlying reasons of the sovereign debt crisis was not consensual, nonetheless. Heterodox approaches to the crisis put the emphasis on current account imbalances between largely indebted member states and another group of countries showing current account surpluses as the trigger of the sovereign debt crisis (Frieden and Walter, 2017).
2 *Financial Times*. 'ECB's Lagarde Urges Governments to Boost Public Investment'. 22 November 2019. Available online at: www.ft.com/content/c3483866-0d07-11ea-b2d6-9bf4d1957a67 [Accessed 23 November 2020].
3 The Guardian. 'Franco-German Plan for European Recovery Will Face Compromises'. 26 May 2020. Available online at: www.theguardian.com/world/2020/may/26/franco-german-plan-for-european-recovery-will-face-compromises [Accessed 23 November 2020].
4 SURE stands for Support to mitigate Unemployment Risks in an Emergency. According to the Commission, 'it will provide financial assistance, in the form of loans granted on favourable terms from the EU to Member States, of up to €100 billion in total' (European Commission, n.d.b).
5 *Politico*. 'European Commission Proposes €750B EU Recovery Package'. 27 May 2020. Available online at: www.politico.eu/article/commission-to-propose-recovery-instrument-of-e750-billion/ [Accessed 23 November 2020].
6 See, for example, Euractive network, 2020. How EU Member States Reacted to the Commission's Recovery Fund Proposal. Available at: www.euractiv.com/section/politics/news/how-eu-member-states-reacted-to-the-commissions-recovery-fund-proposal/ [Accessed 24 November 2020].
7 DW.com. 'European Commission Unveils 750-billion Recovery Plan'. Available at: www.dw.com/en/european-commission-unveils-750-billion-recovery-plan/a-53584998 [Accessed 24 November 2020].

Bibliography

Ambrocio, G., 2020. European Household and Business Expectations during Covid-19: Towards a V-Shaped Recovery in Confidence? *Bank of Finland Economics Review*, No. 27461 [online] Available at: https://helda.helsinki.fi/bof/bitstream/handle/123456789/17538/BoFER_6_2020.pdf?sequence=1&isAllowed=y [Accessed 27 November 2020].

Artis, M. J. and Buti, M., 2000. 'Close-to-Balance or in Surplus': A Policy-Maker's Guide to the Implementation of the Stability and Growth Pact. *Journal of Common Market Studies*, 38(4), pp. 563–91.

Barbieri Góes, M. C. and Gallo, E., 2020. A Predatory-Prey Model of Unemployment and W-shaped Recession in the COVID-19 Pandemic. *No. 2006, Working Papers, New School for Social Research, Department of Economics* [online] Available at: www.economicpolicyresearch.org/econ/2020/NSSR_WP_062020.pdf [Accessed 26 November 2020].

Barrero, J. M., Bloom, N. and Davis, S. J., 2020. COVID-19 Is Also a Reallocation Shock. *NBER Working Paper,* No. 23137 [online] Available at: www.nber.org/papers/w27137 [Accessed 15 November 2020].

Bartik, A. W. et al., 2020. The Impact of COVID-19 on Small Business Outcomes and Expectations. *Proceedings of the National Academy of Sciences of the United States of America*, [e-journal] 117(30), pp. 17656–66. https://doi.org/10.1073/pnas.2006991117.

Benmelehc, E. and Tzur-Ilan, N., 2020. The Determinants of Monetary and Fiscal Policies during the COVID-19 Crisis. *NBER Working Paper*, No. 27461 [online] Available at: www.nber.org/system/files/working_papers/w27461/w27461.pdf [Accessed 17 November 2020].

Borio, C., 2020. The Covid-19 Economic Crisis: Dangerously Unique. *Business Economics*, [e-journal] 55, pp. 181–90. https://doi.org/10.1057/s11369-020-00184-2.

BVerfG, 2020. Headnotes to the Judgment of the Second Senate of 5 May 2020 – 2 BvR 859/15, paras. *1–237*. [online] Available at: www.bverfg.de/e/rs20200505_2bvr085915en.html [Accessed 24 November 2020].

Carlsson-Szlezak, P., Reeves, M. and Swartz, P., 2020. What Coronavirus Could Mean for the Global Economy. *Harvard Business Review* [e-journal], pp. 1–10. Available at: https://hbr.org/2020/03/what-coronavirus-could-mean-for-the-global-economy. [Accessed 27 November 2020].

Casado. M. G. et al., 2020. The Effect of Fiscal Stimulus: Evidence from COVID-19. *NBER Working Paper*, No. 27576 [online] Available at: www.nber.org/system/files/working_papers/w27576/w27576.pdf [Accessed 17 November 2020].

Clift, B., 2020. The Hollowing Out of Monetarism: The Rise of Rules-Based Monetary Policy-Making in the UK and USA and Problems with the Paradigm Change Framework. *Comparative European Politics*, 18, pp. 281–308.

Constantini, O., 2020. The Eurozone as a Trap and a Hostage: Obstacles and Prospects of the Debate on European Fiscal Rules. *Intereconomics: Review of European Economic Policy*, 55(5), pp. 284–91.

De Grauwe, P., 2015. Design failures of the Eurozone. In: R. Baldwin and F. Giavazzi, eds. *The Eurozone Crisis: A Consensus View of the Causes and a Few Possible Remedies*. London: CEPR Press, pp. 99–108.

De Grauwe, P. and Ji, Y., 2019. Time to Change Budgetary Priorities in the Eurozone. *Intereconomics: Review of European Economic Policy*, 54(5), pp. 285–90.

Delatte, A. L. and Guillaume, A., 2020. Covid 19: A New Challenge for the EMU. *CEPR Discussion Paper,* No. DP14848 [online] Available at: https://ssrn.com/abstract=3628168 [Accessed 21 November 2020].

Eichenbaum, M. S., Rebelo, S. and Trabandt, T., 2020. The Macroeconomics of Epidemics, *NBER Working Papers*, No. 26882 [online] Available at: https://ssrn.com/abstract=3562570 [Accessed 14 November 2020].

Eichengreen, B., 2020. Keynesian Economics: Can It Return If It Never Died? *Review of Keynesian Economics*, 8(1), pp. 23–35.

Eurogroup, 2020. Report on the Comprehensive Economic Policy Response to the COVID-19 Pandemic. Available at: www.consilium.europa.eu/pt/press/press-releases/2020/04/09/report-on-the-comprehensive-economic-policy-response-to-the-covid-19-pandemic/. [Accessed 27 November 2020].

European Central Bank, 2020a. Pandemic Emergency Purchase Programme. [online] Available at: www.ecb.europa.eu/mopo/implement/pepp/html/index.en.html [Accessed 23 November 2020].

European Central Bank, 2020b. Monetary Policy Decisions, 10 December 2020. Available at: www.ecb.europa.eu/press/pr/date/2020/html/ecb.mp201210~8c2778b843.en.html. [Accessed 11 December 2020].

European Commission, n.d.b. *SURE Supporting Member Stares to Help Protecting People in Work and Jobs*. Available at: https://ec.europa.eu/info/sites/info/files/economy-finance/sure_factsheet.pdf. [Accessed 27 November 2020].

European Commission, 2020. *Europe's Moment: Repair and Prepare for the Next Generation*. COM(2020) 456 final. Available at: https://eur-lex.europa.eu/legal-content/EN/TXT/PDF/?uri=CELEX:52020DC0456&from=EN [Accessed 24 November 2020].

European Council/Council of the European Union, 2020a. Conclusions of the President of the European Council following the videoconference of the members of the European Council, 17 March 2020. [online] Available at: www.consilium.europa.eu/en/press/press-releases/2020/03/17/conclusions-by-the-president-of-the-european-council-following-the-video-conference-with-members-of-the-european-council-on-covid-19/ [Accessed 24 November 2020].

European Council/Council of the European Union, 2020b. Conclusions of the President of the European Council following the videoconference of the members of the European Council, 23 April 2020. [online] Available at: www.consilium.europa.eu/en/press/press-releases/2020/04/23/conclusions-by-president-charles-michel-following-the-video-conference-with-members-of-the-european-council-on-23-april-2020/ [Accessed 24 November 2020].

European Council/Council of The European Union, 2020c. Joint statement of the Members of the European Council. Available online at: www.consilium.europa.eu/media/43076/26-vc-euco-statement-en.pdf [Accessed 24 November 2020].

Eurostat, 2020. GDP and Main Components (Output, Expenditure and Income), Gross Domestic Product at Market Prices. Available online at: https://ec.europa.eu/eurostat/web/national-accounts/data/main-tables [Accessed 2 December 2020].

Fabbrini, S., 2013. Intergovernmentalism and Its Limits: Assessing the European Union's Answer to the Euro Crisis. *Comparative Political Studies*, 46(9), pp. 1003–29.

Fana, M. et al., 2020. *The COVID Confinement Measures and EU Labour Markets*. Luxembourg: Publications Office of the European Union, doi: 10.2760/079230, JRC120578. Available at: https://publications.jrc.ec.europa.eu/repository/bitstream/JRC120578/jrc120578_report_covid_confinement_measures_final_updated_good.pdf [Accessed 28 January 2021].

Fernandes, N., 2020. Economic Effects of Coronavirus Outbreak (COVID-19) on the World Economy. *IESE Business School Working Paper*, No. WP-1240-E, [online] Available at: https://ssrn.com/abstract=3557504 [Accessed 11 November 2020].

Frieden, J. and Walter, S., 2017. Understanding the Political Economy of the Eurozone Crisis. *Annual Review of Political Science*, 20, pp. 371–90.

Frieden, J. and Walter, S., 2019. Analyzing Inter-state Negotiations in the Eurozone Crisis and Beyond. *European Union Politics*, 20(1), pp. 134–51.

Gallant, J., Kroft, K., Lange, F. and Notowidigdo, M., 2020. Temporary Unemployment and Labour Market Dynamics During the COVID-19 Recession. *NBER Working Paper,* No. 27924 [online] Available at: www.nber.org/system/files/working_papers/w27924/w27924.pdf [Accessed 9 November 2020].

Giavazzi, F. and Tabellini, G., 2020. Covid Perpetual Eurobonds: Jointly Guaranteed and Supported by the ECB. In: A. Bénassy-Quéré and B. Weder di Mauro, eds. *Europe in the Time of Covid-19*. London: CEPR Press. pp. 235–9.

Giavazzi, F. and Wyplosz, C., 2015. EMU: Old Flaws Revisited. *Journal of European Integration*, 37(7), pp. 723–37.

Goolsbee, A. and Syverson, C., 2020. Fear, Lockdown, and Diversion: Comparing Drivers of Pandemic Economic Decline 2020. *Journal of Public Economics*, [e-journal] 193. https://doi.org/10.1016/j.jpubeco.2020.104311.

Gourinchas, P.-O., Kalemli-Özcan, Ş., Penciakova, V. and Sander, N., 2020. COVID-19 and SME Failures. *CEPR Discussion Paper*, No. DP15323, [online] Available at: https://ssrn.com/abstract=3723512 [Accessed 23 November 2020].

Heipertz, M. and Verdun, A., 2010. *Ruling Europe: The Politics of the Stability and Growth Pact*. Cambridge: Cambridge University Press.

Herzog, B., 2020. Whither Coronabonds? The Past and Future of the EMU in the Coronavirus Pandemic. *Intereconomics: Review of European Economic Policy*, 55(3), pp. 155–9.

Ilzetzki, E., Reinhart, C. M. and Rogoff, K. S., 2020. Will the Secular Decline in Exchange Rate and Inflation Volatility Survive Covid-19? *NBER Working Paper*, No. 28108, [online] Available at: www.nber.org/system/files/working_papers/w28108/w28108.pdf [Accessed 19 November 2020].

Jaravel, X. and O'Connell, M., 2020. Real Time Price Indices: Inflation Spike and Falling Product Variety during the Great Lockdown. *Journal of Public Economics*, [e-journal] 191. https://doi.org/10.1016/j.jpubeco.2020.104270.

Kindleberger, C. P., 2006. *Keynesianism vs. Monetarism and Other Essays in Financial History*. London: George Allen & Unwin.

Kratochvíl, P. and Sychra, Z., 2019. The End of Democracy in the EU? The Eurozone Crisis and the EU's Democratic Deficit. *Journal of European Integration*, 41(2), pp. 169–85.

Li, L., Strahan, P. E. and Zhang, S., 2020. Banks as Lenders of First Resort: Evidence from the COVID-19 Crisis. *The Review of Corporate Finance Studies*, 9(3), pp. 472–500.

Lucchese, M. and Pianta, M., 2020. The Coming Coronavirus Crisis: What Can We Learn? *Intereconomics: Review of European Economic Policy*, 55(2), pp. 98–104.

McKibbin, W. and Roshen, F., 2020. The Economic Impact of COVID-19. In: R. Baldwin and B. Weder di Mauro, eds. *Economics in the Time of COVID-19*. London: CEPR Press. pp. 45–52.

Mitchell, W., 2015. *Eurozone Dystopia: Groupthink and Denial on a Grand Scale*. Cheltenham: Edward Elgar.

Modigliani, F., 1977. The Monetarist Controversy, or, Should we Forsake Stabilization Policies? *American Economic Review*, 67(2), pp. 1–17.

Mody, A., 2018. *EuroTragedy: A Drama in Nine Acts*. Oxford: Oxford University Press.

Paulus, A. and Tasseva, I. V., 2020. Europe through the Crisis: Discretionary Policy Changes and Automatic Stabilizers. *Oxford Bulletin of Economics and Statistics*, 82(4), pp. 864–88.

Sachs, J. D., 2020. COVID-19 and Multilateralism. *Horizons: Journal of International Relations and Sustainable Development*, 16, pp. 30–9 [online] Available at: www.jstor.org/stable/48573747 [Accessed 22 November 2020].

Sheth, J., 2020. Impact of Covid-19 on Consumer Behavior: Will the Old Habits Return or Die? *Journal of Business Research* [e-journal] 117, pp. 280–3. https://doi.org/10.1016/j.jbusres.2020.05.059.

Skidelsky, R., 2020. Economic Recovery in the Age of COVID-19. *Intereconomics*, [e-journal] 55, pp. 345–9. https://doi.org/10.1007/s10272-020-0929-6.

Stiglitz, J., 2013. After the Financial Crisis We Were All Keynesians – But Not for Long Enough. *The Guardian*, 10 October 2013 [online] Available at: www.theguardian.com/business/economics-blog/2013/oct/10/financial-crisis-keynesians-eurozone-recession. [Accessed 27 November 2020].

Susskind, D. and Vines, D., 2020. The Economics of the COVID-19 Pandemic: An Assessment, *Oxford Review of Economic Policy*, 36, Issue Supplement_1, pp. S1–S13. https://doi.org/10.1093/oxrep/graa036.

Tesche, T., 2020. The European Union's Response to the Coronavirus Emergency: An Early Assessment. *LSE 'Europe in Question' Discussion Paper Series,* No. 157. [online] Available at: https://ssrn.com/abstract=3624730. [Accessed 9 November 2020].

Velasco, A., 2020. Are We All Keynesians Again? *Project Syndicate*, 25 August 2020, [online] Available at: www.project-syndicate.org/commentary/states-must-be-insurer-of-last-resort-against-aggregate-risks-by-andres-velasco-2020-08?barrier=accesspaylog. [Accessed 27 November 2020].

Wolcott, E., Ochse, M. G., Kudlyak, M. and Kouchekinia, N. A., 2020. Temporary Layoffs and Unemployment in the Pandemic. *FRBSF Economic Letter,* No. 2020–34, [online] Available at: www.frbsf.org/economic-research/files/el2020-34.pdf [Accessed 25 November 2020].

Wyplosz, C., 2006. European Monetary Union: The Dark Sides of a Major Success. *Economic Policy*, 21(46), pp. 208–61.

4 Security or securitisation

Border controls as a setback for European integration?

4.1 Introduction

Freedom of movement is a paramount principle of European integration. The first general provisions on the subject, which date back to the 1957 Treaty of Rome, were essentially related to the goal of establishing an internal market, covering free movement of workers and freedom of establishment, therefore granting rights to individuals that were employees or service providers. However, the evolution of the integration process gradually dissociated the idea of free movement of persons from this economic precondition, turning it into a truly 'cornerstone of EU citizenship' (Marzocchi, 2020).

The COVID-19 pandemic is not the first crisis that justified the introduction of restrictions to free circulation in the EU. But it is certainly the one that resulted in the most severe limitations to mobility within and outside the EU territory. Border closures, restrictions to circulation, and partial and general lockdowns have profoundly impacted citizens' lives, raising concerns about the respect for their rights. Although the level of public health threat resulting from the severity of the COVID-19 pandemic justifies restrictions on some rights, those restrictions cannot be taken lightly.

The chapter opens the sectoral dimension of the book (also featured in Chapters 5 and 6). The analysis focuses on the measures approved by national authorities regarding the closing of internal borders. The stated purpose was to isolate countries from the propagation of COVID-19. Yet, since free movement of persons is a hallmark of the EU, closing borders has an impact on the idiosyncrasy of European integration. We do not suggest that both aspects are in contradiction, as the rationale of border controls is legitimate from the point of view of the rationale of crisis management. We ask if the legitimate claim for security has once again paved the way to the much challenging path of securitisation. Did the implementation of border controls represent a setback for European integration? The chapter is organised as follows. Section 4.2 briefly reviews the evolution of the freedom of movement, from an economic right to a building block of the European way of life. Section 4.3 analyses the processes of securitisation of the COVID-19 pandemic, assessing the conformity of border closures and other restrictions

DOI: 10.4324/9781003153900-5

to free movement to the EU and international law. Section 4.4 looks at the reverse process of de-securitisation, highlighting the narrative shift. Section 4.5 considers the possibility of change resulting from the lessons learned.

4.2 Freedom of movement as a cornerstone of European citizens' way of life

The earliest provisions on the free movement of persons were laid down in the Treaty of Paris (1951), establishing the European Coal and Steel Community (ECSC), but were limited to the mobility of coal and steel workers. In the subsequent Treaty of Rome (1957), establishing the European Economic Community (EEC), the free movement of workers was one of the four freedoms[1] essential to build the pet project of the Treaty: a European common market. The idea was to guarantee that workers and other economically active persons were allowed to move freely and to establish themselves within the EEC territory, providing that they were capable of supporting themselves in the destination country. Therefore, the right to move freely was intended to apply only to people who were economically active, which in practice excluded many Europeans from this freedom. However, as it frequently happens with the EU legal texts, EEC Treaty dispositions and the implementing secondary legislation, 'left room for interpretation' (Koikkalainen, 2011). EU free movement law has, therefore, steadily advanced through secondary legislation and through the case law of the ECJ, which was a particular interventive actor in this field (Sánchez, 2015). Indeed, the ECJ ruling was instrumental for widening the scope of free movement. One important move was the ECJ's interpretation of the concept of 'worker', which was gradually expanded to include seasonal workers and short-time employment and apprenticeship placements. Eventually, the freedom of movement was extended to students, pensioners, the unemployed, as well as to their families (Koikkalainen, 2011). Also, relevant was the prohibition of any type of discrimination on the grounds of nationality.

Besides the jurisprudential and legislative push, other factors contributed to the transformation of the free-movement rights into a building block of the EU political project, central to the construction of a supranational identity (Sánchez, 2015). Two hallmarks of the EU integration process had a significant impact on the evolution of free movement. The first was the conclusion of the Schengen agreements (including the 1985 Schengen Agreement and the 1990 Convention to implementing the Agreement, that came into force in 1995), which essentially created a common borderless area between the five initial signatories (Belgium, France, Germany, Luxembourg and the Netherlands), through intergovernmental cooperation in the area of justice and home affairs. Shortly after, the so-called 'Schengen acquis' was transferred into the treaties by a Protocol annex to the Amsterdam Treaty (1999). The creation of the Schengen area included, amidst other achievements, (i) the abolition of internal border controls for all persons; (ii) a certain degree of harmonisation of external border controls; (iii) a common visa policy for short stays; (iv) police and judicial cooperation; and (v) the development (and later reinforcement) of the Schengen Information System (SIS) (Marzocchi, 2020). Currently 22 EU member states and four non-EU members states[2] are part of the Schengen area, resulting that, in practice, European citizens are free to cross the majority of intra-European borders without having to stop at border controls. Although the Schengen area is a remarkable success, several events raised considerable challenges, namely the terrorist attacks that have occurred in some EU member states over the last two decades, the migration crisis and now the ongoing COVID-19 pandemic.

The other milestone was the introduction of the EU citizenship (thought to complement national citizenship) in the Treaty of Maastricht. The legal roots of a European citizenship could be found precisely in the free movement of workers' provisions of the EEC Treaty. Although initially connected to the common market, labour mobility encompassed from the start the embryo of a European citizenship. Indeed, as workers were able to invoke and exercise free movement rights independently of the approval of host member states, this could be considered an 'incipient form of EU citizenship', although reserved 'for certain classes of persons, that is, workers, professionals, service providers, and their families' (Kostakopoulou, 2013, p. 20). The idea of a common European citizenship was developed during the 1970s and the 1980s through initiatives such as the European Identity Declaration (1973), the first direct elections for the EP (1979), the Commission's proposals regarding residence or electoral rights of Community nationals inhabiting in host member states, the introduction of the first uniform passport (1981) or the recommendation for formal establishment of a EU citizenship by the Draft Treaty on the European Union approved by the EP in 1984 (Kostakopoulou, 2013, pp. 20–21). This evolution culminated in the formal introduction of EU citizenship by the Treaty of Maastricht. Whereas the new European citizenship added new rights to the existing free movement and residence rights, the later remained at the very core of the new status. Actually, this is one fundamental difference in relation to national citizenships: '[w]hile national citizenships presuppose peoples' rootedness, EU citizenship has been intimately linked to citizens' mobility and to border crossings'[3] (Kostakopoulou, 2013, p. 14). In the following decade, another fundamental EU text, the EU Charter of Fundamental Rights also provided for freedom of movement and residence in its Article 45.

By explicitly evolving from free movement of *workers* to free movement of *persons*, freedom of movement became a foundation of a European way of life. However, it also became one of the most 'complex and challenging of the EU freedoms, both legally and politically' (Cuyvers, 2017, p. 354). It is directly linked with many other EU policy areas such as the internal market, but also social security, immigration, healthcare, public order or information collecting and sharing, therefore limiting the room for the exercise of member states' autonomy in those areas.

4.3 Dilemmas of COVID-19 securitisation

Security is commonly perceived as a fundamental value for people. In the academia, security studies gained prominence in the aftermath of the World War II as a subfield of International Relations (IR). Consequently, security studies were influenced by the dominant, state-centric, IR paradigm at the time, Realism, which emphasised state's survival in the anarchic international system. The research agenda was mainly concerned with the protection of the state from definable threats (for the most part military threats) and the preservation of the status quo. This 'traditionalist' view of security (Buzan, Waever and de Wilde, 1998) was challenged by the Copenhagen School (through the works of Ole Waever, Barry Buzan, Jaap de Wilde, and others), which approached security through a social constructivist lens, laying the basis of wider securitisation studies. The main goal was to extend the research agenda beyond the 'traditional' military context, to include new, often nonmilitary, sources of threat that came from other sectors: political, economic, societal and environmental security. The authors also intended to broaden the referent object for security to objects other than the state, by including individuals, socials groups and the international society. Rather than an objective (or subjective) condition, for the Copenhagen School security has a discursive and political nature embedded and is a concept that does something – to securitise. Thus, securitisation refers to the process of presenting an issue in security terms, that is, as an existential threat (Buzan and Hansen, 2009, p. 214):

> [i]f by means of an argument about the priority and urgency of an existential threat the securitizing actor has managed to break free of procedures or rules he or she would otherwise be bound by, we are witnessing a case of securitization.
>
> (Buzan, Waever and de Wilde, 1998, p. 25)

Considering this line of reasoning, once an issue is securitised by securitising agents (usually political leaders, bureaucracies, governments, lobbyists and pressure groups), it ceases to be debated as a political question and starts to be 'dealt with at an accelerated pace and in ways that may violate normal legal and social rules' (Buzan, Waever and de Wilde, 1998, p. 23). To put it differently:

> once something is securitized, then normal/political means and actions are replaced by security concerns, and extraordinary protection measures can be imposed, and easily justified, without ever being questioned.
>
> (Vankovska, 2020, p. 74)

The COVID-19 pandemic is clearly illustrative of this securitisation process. In EU member states, and in many countries worldwide, the disease was presented in security terms, portrayed by national leaders as a clear threat to the state and citizens. What is more, the use of 'war-like rhetoric against the invisible enemy' (Vankovska, 2020, p. 73) was adopted by many political leaders,[4] journalists and members of the scientific community. The utilisation of metaphors, such as war metaphors, to describe complex problems is not uncommon, as they allow people to 'talk and think about complex or abstract information in terms of comparatively simple and more concrete information' (Flusberg, Matlock and Thibodeau, 2018, p. 6). For the authors, war metaphors are effective in communication because there is a clear understanding of what war involves (a fight against an enemy, strategic decisions, a hierarchy of command and events, a sense of urgency and risk); this knowledge is widespread (wars are an important part of human experience); many common topics of discussion resemble war, as they structure relations and can evoke similar emotions (e.g., the idea of a virus as a foreign invader of the body); as a result of the former three, they are prevalent in communication, that is, they are familiar because they are frequently used (Flusberg, Matlock and Thibodeau, 2018, pp. 9–10). Nevertheless, we must note that the resource to war metaphors to describe the COVID-19 pandemic has not been widely accepted,[5] with opponents alerting for the potential perils of using this comparison, that included 'creating excessive anxiety, potentially legitimizing authoritarian governmental measures, and implying that those who die did not fight hard enough' (Semino, 2021, p. 50). The widespread use of war metaphors in various situations in various societies suggests they have a resonance owing to their ability to simplify complex issues, improve communication, capture attention and motivate action.

In the twenty-first century, two apparently opposite narratives seem to coexist on securitisation. On the one hand, many agree that in globalised world new forms of global health governance that supersede state-centric approaches are needed to find a solution to infectious diseases outbreaks. Diseases certainly do not stop at borders and therefore international cooperation is the key to effective responses. On the other hand, in a process of securitisation, governments have increasingly come to see public health problems as national security threats, meaning that 'we have a national security framing of disease threats in which defending the nation (and therefore its borders) has taken on a new level of importance' (Ferhani and Rushton, 2020, p. 459). Arguably, thus, the securitisation process helped to legitimise the severe restrictions governments imposed on citizens, clearly limiting rights that are at the core of national and European citizenships, such as the freedom of movement.

Confronted with the rapid spread of the SARS-CoV-2 virus in Europe, EU countries, as many others outside the EU, reacted by adopting a traditional 'self-help' stance and by unilaterally deciding the introduction of internal border controls and travel restrictions.[6] Actually, this type of response was not a novelty, as indeed border closures and restrictions on foreign travellers 'have been the most persistent and pervasive means by which states have responded to global health crises' (Kenwick and Simmons, 2020, p. E36). Eventually,

EU external borders were also subject to severe restrictions to travelling from and to the EU: '[r]estrictions on international and intra-EU traffic of persons has become one of the most visible policy responses to the Coronavirus pandemic' (Carrera and Luk, 2020, p. 14). The decision to close external borders granted the EU criticisms from external partners: '[t]he move ruffled feathers among Europe's partners, some of which had lower infection rates than the EU' (Mortera-Martinez, 2020, p. 2).

The closing of borders was paired with confinement measures applied in the territory of each EU country that strongly impacted on free movement of persons but also in other citizens' rights. All member states have, to some degree, prohibited public gatherings (or imposed limits to the number of people that could meet in public and private spaces), closed schools and shops, cancelled public events, declared the shutdown of activities considered non-essential (such as leisure, hotel and restaurant activities) and dictated partial or full lockdowns. Many of them have also proclaimed a state of emergency (see Chapter 6). The justification for adopting such restrictive measures was to halt the spread of the virus. Therefore, member states' initial concern appeared to be self-preservation, that is, to guarantee the security of their population. This is a normal reaction from states shaken with a severe external security threat (Deen and Kruijver, 2020) and confirms the idea that the COVID-19 issue was securitised.

This inward-looking type of response casted serious doubts on the utility of the EU membership and on the true meaning of EU solidarity (see Chapter 2). However, from a constitutional stance, it seems reasonable that member states act to protect their population against a serious threat and therefore decide both the level of health protection needed and the measures to put it in place, including restrictions on mobility (Berrod and Bruyas, 2020). As a matter of fact, human rights law recognise that under certain contexts (including serious public health threats or public emergencies threatening the life of a nation) restrictions on some rights might be justified, provided certain conditions are fulfilled:

> [to] have a legal basis, are strictly necessary, based on scientific evidence and neither arbitrary nor discriminatory in application, of limited duration, respectful of human dignity, subject to review, and proportionate to achieve the objective.
>
> (Human Rights Watch, 2020)

Furthermore, within the EU framework of governance, Articles 25 to 30 of the Schengen Borders Code (SBC) allow member states to introduce internal border controls, provided the measures are decided 'as a last resort', are 'temporary' and proportional in relation to the threat (Article 26 of SBC). The decision on whether to introduce restrictions to free movement to protect the state against a serious threat thus remains a prerogative of EU member states. It is worth noting that the SBC only explicitly mentions public health threats as a justification to implement controls at external borders regarding third-country nationals (Articles 6. and 8 of SBC). Regardless of the justification, the Commission and the other member states have to be notified of the decision, the reasons and the scope of the proposed reintroduction of border controls, as well as the date and duration of the planned reintroduction (Article 26 of SBC). Article 28 of the SBC opens the door to immediate reintroduction of border controls at internal borders in case of 'serious threat to public policy or internal security in a Member State [that] requires immediate action'.

Thus, these measures are limited to a period up to 10 days (renewable for periods up to 20 days, with a limitation of 2–18 months, depending on the seriousness and persistence of the threat) and did not exempt the member state of notifying the Commission and the other member states (the notification must occur at the same time of the reintroduction of border controls) (Article 29 of SBC). Thus, although allowing the reintroduction of border controls, the SBC puts on member states 'the burden of proof to substantiate and justify the necessity and proportionality of any border and travel restrictions derogating free movement' (Carrera and Luk, 2020, p. 49). Also, the emphasis on the proportionality of the measures adopted implies that member states are obliged to permanently reassess the pertinence and effectiveness of the reintroduction of border controls, particularly as these measures negatively impact on EU citizen's rights and freedoms. It should be noted that besides the provisions laid down in the SBC, any restriction on the freedom of movement has to comply with EU free movement rules envisaged in the Treaties and in secondary legislation,[7] some of which, such as the so-called Citizens' Directive, has explicit reference to public health issues as grounds to restrict the freedom of movement.[8]

As regards the EU formal procedures, despite a rocky start,[9] the majority of member states respected formal procedures and followed the dispositions of the SBC as regards notification requirements of border closures on the grounds of COVID-19.[10] However, questions remain on whether member states made an 'opportunistic' use of the idea of serious threat to public policy and internal security. For Carrera and Luk (2020) member states had indeed an 'instrumental' approach to the COVID-19 pandemic:

> the key assessment role attributed to border and police authorities results in a disproportionate degree of discretion regarding what the legitimate set of grounds are for justifying border controls or equivalent travel restrictions.
>
> (Carrera and Luk, 2020, p. 57)

As regards other conditions required by the EU and the international law, although, in principle, restrictions on free movement might also conform with it, several questions arise from the disruption of citizens' rights in face of the pandemic. The immediate question, related to the precondition of clear *necessity* based on scientific evidence, is whether border closures is an effective way to protect public health. Grépin et al. (2020) made a systematic review of studies aimed at assessing the effectiveness of travel-related measures (such as screening, travel restrictions and border closures) to halt the outbreak of influenza and other infectious diseases, including COVID-19. Although some studies on previous influenza epidemics and pandemics have found some evidence that border closures could delay the arrival and the spread of the epidemic, the overall size of the effects was considered relatively small. Also, the timing of the introduction of borders restrictions is key, as the effect on the delay of spread of the virus is greatly reduced when restrictions were imposed several weeks after the onset of an epidemic (Grépin et al., 2020, p. 5).

Regarding the COVID-19 pandemic, the majority of the studies endorsed the idea that the adoption of travel measures let to a positive change in the dynamics of the early phases of the pandemic (even though the results were mainly related to initial export of cases out of Wuhan and just a few concerned the effectiveness of measures adopted in other contexts). One idea that is consensual is that early implementation of travel-related measures is a determinant of effectiveness (Grépin et al., 2020, p. 2). However, as one of the studies reviewed explained, travel limitations have only a modest effect unless paired with public health interventions and behavioural changes that can facilitate a considerable reduction in the transmissibility of the disease (Chinazzi et al., 2020, p. 6). Zanin and Papo (2020) also conducted a study that investigated the effects of travel restrictions during pandemics. The effectiveness of travel restriction measures requires two important pre-requisites: the nonexistence of cases in the isolated territory (a condition difficult to guarantee especially when dealing with a disease that has asymptomatic cases); and travel bans should be total to avoid cross-territory spreading (Zanin and Papo, 2020, p. 2). Using a simulation model, the authors assessed the effects of unidirectional mobility from larger cities to smaller towns during the pandemic. Overall, they concluded that although travel restrictions are beneficial for regions that have a low infection rate (since the new imported cases are limited), this, nevertheless, 'goes against the interest of the system as a whole, as free movements can reduce the total number of cases' (Zanin and Papo, 2020, p. 1).

Arguably, the conclusions highlighted above show that the current scientific evidence is not sufficient to support the absolute necessity of border closures. Also, it was unclear if the lessons from other types of infectious disease outbreaks would be relevant in the context of the COVID-19 pandemic. The scientific evidence at the time might therefore explain the WHO's decision to not recommend travel restrictions when it declared COVID-19 a Public Health Emergency of International Concern (Grépin et al., 2020). It thus seems fair to argue that, in the face of the unknown, states reached for the well-known tools through which they can rapidly assert authority, that is, the control at territorial borders (Kenwick and Simmons, 2020, p. E38). To sum up:

> [t]he ubiquity of these policies is not driven by any clear scientific consensus about their utility in the face of myriad pandemic threats. Instead it is a reflection of their palliative impact on societies predisposed to express concern about that which is foreign in times of crisis.
>
> (Kenwick and Simmons, 2020, p. E36)

Another issue worthy of reflection is whether the measures adopted by member states match with the principles of proportionality and non-discrimination described in the EU treaties and also in the international law. Although restrictions on mobility was a strategy shared by the majority of European countries, the scale, stringency and pace of those measures greatly varied across EU member states (Sabat et al., 2020; International Monetary Fund, 2020; Fana et al., 2020; Lang, 2021). Whereas some governments (such as Spain, Italy, France or Portugal) decided to impose severe limitations on population movements, others adopted lesser rigid measures or no confinement at all (Sabat et al., 2020). The variations in the rates of transmissibility and the number of people infected between EU countries and even between regions within one country might explain disparities regarding the severity of restrictions to mobility and their length.

However, studies that have assessed the proportionality of the measures imposing restrictions to mobility during the first wave of the pandemic raised serious doubts regarding the capacity of member states to enforce and monitor internal border checks and intra- and extra-EU travel bans and other restrictions on mobility. These studies also raised doubts regarding member states' ability to comply with the 'burden of proof', that is, the ability to clearly demonstrate (based on scientific evidence) that the measures were proportional to the threat (Carrera and Luk, 2020, p. 70). Actually, these concerns are not limited to the measures implemented during the pandemic's first wave, but extended to the subsequent reintroduction of border closures in the face of an increase of infection rates. Illustrative of these doubts is the letter of warning that the Commission sent to six EU countries (Belgium, Denmark, Finland, Germany, Hungary and Sweden) on 23 February 2021. According to a Commission's spokesman cited by Euronews, the letter pointed to a risk of 'fragmentation and disruptions to free movement and to supply chains' (Amiel, 2021). It was also asserted that the measures imposed by these countries were disproportional and unjustified.[11]

As for the principle of non-discrimination, the balance is mixed at best. Several EU countries fail to apply entry restrictions equally to all EU citizens. Also, some member states have adopted entry restrictions that differentiate between their own nationals and residents and other EU citizens. Although one might argue that this 'discrimination by design' (Carrera and Luk, 2020, p. 71) is a result of the differences in the severity of the pandemic in each state, it clearly contradicts the EU Treaties' provisions that prohibit any discrimination on the grounds of nationality. Furthermore, this discrimination inevitably impacted on the process of *othering*, that is, the negative distinction between *our group* and the *others*:

> [n]ew bordering practices separate residents from nonresidents, the quarantined from the unquarantined, and the healthy from the unhealthy, while the reinforcement of longer-standing national and local borders galvanizes territorial identities.
>
> (Liu and Bennett, 2020, p. 161)

When assessed through the broader lens of fundamental rights (of which the principle of non-discrimination is an integrant part), the closing of borders raises important questions, particularly as regards the right of refugees to access protection and asylum procedures (Ramji-Nogales and Lang, 2020; Chetail, 2020). Although this debate is beyond the scope of the present chapter, this is a crucial discussion, particularly to prevent that states are able to 'instrumentally' use the COVID-19 threat to restrict migration flows, disregarding migrants and refuges' fundamental rights. As Chetail (2020, p. 5) noted, '[i]nternational human rights law draws a clear-cut dividing line between what states can do and what they must do to protect public health at their borders.' Furthermore, if we extend the exercise to restrictions of free movement other than border closures, a fruitful line of research would be to analyse if some EU member states have capitalised on the pandemic to restrict civic freedoms beyond what was necessary.[12] Chapter 6 explores this issue.

4.4 Reopen Europe: de-securitisation in place?

If political elites often use the process of securitisation to justify potentially unpopular measures, the opposite process – de-securitisation – occurs when they wish to take an issue from the heightened discourse of security, bringing it back to the space of political deliberation (Murphy, 2021). The de-securitisation process thus entails (re)framing COVID-19 from a security threat to a 'manageable situation' suitable to public policy interventions and, as occurred with the opposite dynamic (securitisation), it played out in the news and social media, in the debates between the expert community (Sears, 2020) and in the speeches and other communications of political leaders.

Following a decline of infection transmission rates, most Schengen countries started to lift their internal border controls from around mid-May 2020 (Carrera and Luk, 2020). The lift was coordinated by the Commission, which defined the parameters for the gradual reopening. On 13 April 2020, the President of the Commission and the President of the European Council issued a *Joint European Roadmap towards Lifting COVID-19 Containment Measures*. The document served two purposes: to prepare 'an exit strategy' coordinated with member states from the restrictive measures imposed by member states to stop the spread of the virus and to 'prepare the ground for a comprehensive recovery plan and unprecedented investment' (Von der Leyen and Michel, 2020, p. 1). Although recognising that there was a long way to go, the document de-securitised the threat by pointing out the goal of returning to *normality* and by putting a sort of expiration date on extraordinary measures (that should be progressively substituted by general measures): '[e]ven though the way back to normality will be very long, it is also clear that the extraordinary confinement measures cannot last indefinitely' (Von der Leyen and Michel, 2020, p. 3). The idea that the lifting was justified to guarantee the regular working of the SM was also implicit[13] (as the document noted that the restrictive measures seriously affected the functioning of the SM) (p. 2, 4, 11).

The document thus provided a set of recommendations to member states for a gradual unwinding of travel restrictions and controls at internal borders, taking into consideration epidemiological criteria, health system capacity and appropriate monitoring capacity. In a communication[14] issued on 13 May 2020, while acknowledging that temporary border controls were aimed at delaying the spread of the virus and to reduce this risk of excessive pressure on health care systems, the Commission again emphasised the idea of normal life, noting that 'Europe's societies and economies have to go back to a normal state of functioning' (European Commission, 2020a, p. 2). For the institution this it was time to 'return to the unrestricted free movement of persons and restoring the integrity of the Schengen area, one of the major achievements of European integration' (European Commission, 2020a, p. 1) To support the proposal, the Commission recalled that '[r]estricting free movement and reintroducing internal borders harm the Single Market (…). More than this, they harm our European way of life (…)' (European Commission, 2020a, p. 2).

By the same token, in a meeting held on 5 June 2020, Home Affairs ministers recognised the need to move towards lifting some of the measures that have been applied at national or regional level, including the gradual lifting of border controls and the return to the free movement of persons, which has been limited due to the pandemic.[15] A few days later (11 June 2020), the Commission confirmed that the lifting of travel restrictions and internal border controls was 'firmly underway' (European Commission, 2020b, p. 7) and advised the coordinated lifting of the restrictions at the EU external border, considering the 'continuous positive trend within the EU+ area with regard to the epidemiological situation' (European Commission, 2020b, p. 2). On 15 July 2020, the Commission adopted a communication dubbed *Short-Term EU Health Preparedness for COVID-19 Outbreaks*, aimed at increasing the level of preparation of the EU for possible new waves of the disease:

> [l]earning the lessons of the earlier stages of the pandemic, Europe must use this period of lower transmission rates to reinforce its preparedness and coordinated response capacity to counter further outbreaks of COVID-19.
>
> (European Commission, 2020c, p. 1)

Besides several recommendations directly related to health and the health sector,[16] the document included a section on non-pharmaceutical countermeasures. On this subject, the document highlighted the negative economic and social impact of large-scale lockdown measures, advising against its use. Rather, the document recommended that the response 'should be to have targeted and localised non-medical countermeasures, informed by research and evidence' (European Commission, 2020c, p. 10). The document also discouraged the reintroduction of EU internal border controls, and more generally, the adoption of measures that imply restrictions on the movement of persons and goods, unless it was absolutely essential.

From mid-June 2020 onwards, the idea of gradually returning economic and social life to 'normality' across Europe dominated the EU narrative. Lifting border controls and restoring free movement was found essential. The disruptive economic and social impact of the restrictions was recurrently highlighted, meaning that:

> [t]he reestablishment of ineffective restrictions and internal EU border controls must be avoided moving forward. Any measures that imply restrictions on the movement of persons or goods within the EU should be used only in situations where it is strictly necessary.
>
> (European Commission, 2020f, p. 10)

Instead, it was repeatedly emphasised the need to strengthen Europe's level of preparedness and response in case of resurgence of COVID-19 outbreaks, using both medical and non-medical countermeasures. For example, the EU vaccine strategy (see Chapters 2 and 5) was envisaged as instrumental to the return to 'normality' across Europe (European Commission, 2020f, p. 7). The development and support of the use of interoperable contact-tracing apps was another example. The EU supported the development of a common approach to using data and digital applications, such as contact-tracing mobile applications, in the response to the coronavirus crisis, namely by supporting health authorities at the national and EU level in monitoring and containing the pandemic (European Commission, 2020e, p. 8). As of November 2020, a total of 23 member states developed or endorsed contact-tracing apps to help halting the spreading of the virus (Dumbrava, 2020, p. 8), although public adherence to the initiative was generally modest (Hernández-Quevedo et al., 2020). In Portugal, for example, as of November 2020, the Stayaway Covid app (that was made available from 1 September 2020) had more than 2.5 million downloads but the number of codes inserted (each infected person receives a code that needs to be introduced in the application) was roughly 1.300 (out of the 4.485 that were issued).[17]

This 'back to normality' turn also implied that other dimensions of the crisis, namely the socio-economic one, were prioritised. A return to a totally operative Schengen area was therefore crucial. The idea was clear in a European Parliament resolution (June 2020):

> [W]hereas a return to a fully functional Schengen area is of the utmost importance to safeguard the principle of freedom of movement as one of the main achievements of European integration and as a key prerequisite for the EU's economic recovery after the COVID-19 pandemic.
>
> (European Parliament, 2020, p. 3)

The European Council, in a special meeting in July 2020, also acknowledged that:

> *We are slowly exiting the acute health crisis. While utmost vigilance is still required on the sanitary situation, the emphasis is now shifting to mitigating the socio-economic damage.*
>
> (European Council, 2020, p. 1, italics in the original)

However, as early as August 2020, the number of COVID-19 cases started to increase across much of the EU. As a response to the new surge of infections, some member states began to reinstate restrictions to free movement. Despite the setback, the EU narrative did not fundamentally change. The message conveyed by EU institutions maintained that any restrictions to free movement should be used as a last resort and should be applied in compliance with the general principles of EU law, namely proportionality and non-discrimination. In order to avoid uncoordinated, unilateral actions, the emphasis was on guaranteeing that any measures with an impact on EU citizens' rights to move and reside freely within the territory of the member states would be coordinated at the EU level:

> The COVID-19 pandemic has disrupted our daily lives in many ways. Travel restrictions have made it difficult for some of our citizens to get to work, to university or to visit their loved ones (…) It is our common duty to ensure coordination on any measures which affect free movement and to give our citizens all the information they need when deciding on their travel.
>
> (Roth, cited in Petrequin, 2020)

The idea of a coordinated response at the EU level was hardly new. In fact, since March 2020 the Commission insisted on a coordinated response in the various dimensions of the pandemic and adopted several guidelines and communications with the aim of supporting coordination efforts of member states, including as regards safeguarding the free movement within the Union in times of the COVID-19 pandemic. Other EU institutions have also endorsed the idea of coordinated action (see Chapter 2). However, by the time the possibility of a second wave of the pandemic was looming on the horizon the lessons from the first responses to the COVID-19 crisis were clear. During the first wave of the pandemic, member states engaged in a 'self-help approach' that ultimately hindered the effectiveness of the measures adopted and casted some doubts on their compliance with EU law and international law. The securitisation of the public health problem at the early stages of the crisis helped to diffuse the criticisms, enabling for measures to be adopted without a clear scientific assessment of their absolute necessity to the solution:

> Member States have provided little justification in their formal notifications under the Schengen Borders Code as to how border control is an appropriate means to limit the spread of COVID-19.
>
> (European Parliament, 2020, p. 3)

However, as the COVID-19 problem was de-securitised, a more thoughtful assessment of the measures implemented would naturally follow. For instance, the need to find clear and objective criteria, based on scientific evidence, to adopt measures that have an impact on citizens' rights became pivotal. Thus, at the beginning of September 2020, the Commission issued a proposal for a Council recommendation on a coordinated approach to the restriction of free movement in response to the COVID-19 pandemic, stating that '[r]estoring freedom of movement, while protecting public health, is a priority (…)' (European Commission, 2020g, p. 1).

The Council adopted the recommendation on 12 October 2020,[18] determining that any measures must be proportionate and not discriminatory and must be lifted as soon as the epidemiological situation allows. The recommendation also established the key points of the coordinated approach, namely: (i) the application of common criteria and thresholds for the eventual introduction of restrictions to free movement; (ii) a mapping of the risk of COVID-19 transmission based on an agreed colour code published by the ECDC; and (iii) a coordinated approach to eventual measures restricting mobility between areas (depending on the level of risk of transmission in those areas) (Council of the European Union, 2020b, p. 6). The maps published by the ECDC every Thursday that divided regions in colours depending on infection rates (based on the data reported by EU member states to the European Surveillance System database) are a result of this Recommendation.[19] Confirming that, although the epidemiological situation was deteriorating in some member states, the 'return to normality' narrative was upheld, the document explicitly mentioned that:

> [t]his Recommendation should not be understood as facilitating or encouraging the adoption of restrictions to free movement put in place in response to the pandemic, but rather seeks to provide a coordinated approach in the event that a Member State were to decide to introduce such restrictions.
>
> (Council of the European Union, 2020b, p. 6).

Eventually though, all EU member states experienced a second and third waves of the pandemic. Epidemiologists point to a combination of reasons for the new surges, including a relaxation of lockdowns, public's loosening of precautionary behaviour (Looi, 2020) and the appearance of more transmissible new strains of the virus. The second wave (and afterwards the third) was more evenly spread than the first (*The Economist*, 2020), even if there were cross-country differences in the pace of new infections. Thus, though reluctantly, political leaders across Europe had again to impose partial or full lockdowns and border controls. But the 'pandemic fatigue' and the process of de-securitisation that supported the idea of reopening Europe (in June 2020) would require that the purpose of the new regional and national shutdowns was clearly articulated, which was not always the case (*The Economist*, 2020). The result was that protests have broken out in several EU countries, such as Germany, Italy and Spain (*The Economist*, 2020).

Despite the new restrictions on free movement, the EU narrative still emphasised the importance of the right to move freely within the EU as 'one of the EU's most cherished achievements, and an important driver of its economy' (European Commission, 2021, p. 1). Therefore, the emphasis was on measures that facilitate free movement, while guaranteeing protection against the health threat. One example was the proposal for a Digital Green Certificate framework that may include vaccination certificates as well other certificates issued during the COVID-19 pandemic (namely documents certifying a negative test result for SARS-CoV-2 infection as well as documents certifying that the person concerned has recovered from a previous infection) in order to facilitate the exercise of free movement (European Commission, 2021, p. 3).

4.5 Lessons from the COVID-19 pandemic: the 'pandemicisation' of border controls and the idea of security over freedom?

Over the last year, we have witnessed a successive on and off of measures restricting free movement, including internal and external border controls. This intermittence makes it difficult to clearly assess if and how pandemic related measures, namely border closures, altered the fundamental nature of freedom of movement in the long run. A clear peril relates to the difficult balance between security and freedom. Indeed, the COVID-19 pandemic has highlighted 'the challenges in finding the right balance between disease control and protection of fundamental freedoms, and between the level of health risks and societal risk tolerance' (Lang, 2021, p. 24).

One possible angle to approach this question is to see how citizens perceived and assessed the measures adopted by the governments of member states, particularly as some measures highlighted the importance of security at the expense of freedom. According to a poll conducted by the European Council on Foreign Relations at the height of COVID-19 in Europe (covering nine EU member states[20]), a substantial share of the respondents supported the idea of stricter border controls (ranging from 48 per cent in Denmark to 73 per cent in Portugal) (Zerka, 2020). Before concluding that this represents a profound shift in the way EU citizens value their freedom of movement, these results should be analysed together with responses to other questions. Indeed, when asked if the EU should have more control over external and internal borders once the pandemic is over, the percentage of respondents that answer favourably was higher regarding external borders (ranging from 33 per cent in Italy to 61 per cent in Bulgaria), than regarding internal borders (only a minority, ranging from 26 per cent in Italy to 48 per cent in Portugal supported the idea) (Zerka, 2020). Furthermore, this apparently large acceptance of border restrictions might be circumstantial, resulting both from the deep sense of vulnerability that a global crisis without a clear end entails and from the perception that limits on free movement is a necessary part of dealing with a crisis with these characteristics (Zerka, 2020).

A different poll, conducted by the Pew Research Center between 10 June and 3 August 2020, surveyed eight EU member states.[21] The poll showed that the majority of the respondents agreed with their state handling of the pandemic, ranging from 48 per cent in Spain to a remarkable 95 per cent in Denmark (Silver et al., 2020, p. 22). Yet, as the crisis evolved and the pandemic entered the second and the third waves, citizens became less supportive of the restrictions and the level of protests become stronger:

> civil society intensified its response and fought back, often stepping in when governments went beyond what was necessary and proportionate to fight the public health crisis.
>
> (Narsee, 2021, p. 1)

One different, but related question has to do with the idea of unity. As Kenwick and Simmons noted, some publics and politicians focused on a narrative of 'dangerous others' (2020, p. E42). Bordering practices during the pandemic exponentiated divisions, by underlining national and local borders and stimulating territorial identities. Arguably, one legitimate concern is whether this territorial mentality could jeopardise the existence of an area without border controls, such as the Schengen area. Even though there are no indications that these border closures and travel bans will become permanent, some 'pandemicisation' (Ramón, 2020) of borders' governance (including traveller screenings and some travel restrictions) is a possibility, raising concerns about the crisis-proof nature of the Schengen area.

Recent past experiences confirm this as, for example, six member states have maintained border controls since the migration crisis of 2015 (Bossong, 2020; Montaldo, 2020), and France has checks in place since the 2015 Paris terrorist attacks (Mortera-Martinez, 2020). On a positive note, however, the pandemic and the fragilities it showed could be seen as a window of opportunity to a long due reform of the Schengen agreement. Indeed, concerns about the functioning of the Schengen area predated the pandemic by at least one decade and include unresolved questions regarding 'old problems', such as cross-border security, terrorism or irregular migration (Dumbrava, 2020).

The calls for reform have been frequent. In 2017, acting on those calls, the Juncker Commission submitted a proposal to amend the SBC. The main goal was to extend time limits for temporary reintroduction of border controls (up to one year instead of six months) and the limit for the length of prolongation periods (from up to 30 days to up to six months), while introducing additional procedural safeguards (European Commission, 2017, p. 3). The proposal is yet to be agreed upon by the co-legislators (Dumbrava, 2020) and is currently awaiting the Council's first reading.

The current public health threat reopened the debate about the Schengen reform. One of the lessons learned is that countries need to cooperate more effectively on early warning and risk assessment (Erzen et al., 2020). Also, an effective oversight of the health emergency-related use of Articles 25 and 28 of the SBC is crucial (Montaldo, 2020). In June 2020, the EP urged member states (in the Council) and the Commission to discuss a Recovery Plan for Schengen 'in order to prevent temporary internal border controls from becoming semi-permanent in the medium term' (European Parliament, 2020, p. 5). On 23 September 2020, the Commission presented a New Pact on Migration and Asylum (and a Road Map to implement the Pact), where it recognised that the Schengen area has been 'under strain by difficulties in responding to changing situations at the Union's border, by gaps and loopholes, and by diverging national asylum, reception and return systems' (European Commission, 2020d, p. 14). Thus, building on the experience from multiple crises of the last five years, the Commission promised to present a Strategy on the Future of Schengen, including a reform of the SBC, an improvement of the Schengen evaluation mechanism and the establishment of a dedicated Schengen Forum involving the relevant national authorities (such as ministers of home affairs and border police) in order to stimulate concrete cooperation and trust (European Commission, 2020h, pp. 14–15). Interestingly enough, the new Strategy on the Future of Schengen appears under the subtitle 'Promoting Our European Way of Life' in the Commission Work Programme 2021 (European Commission, 2020i, p. 6).

The first meeting of the Schengen Forum (with the presence of home affairs ministers, the president of the Commission, Commission vice-president Margaritis Schinas and the commissioner for home affairs, Ylva Johansson) was held on 30 November 2020. During the event, the intention of an overhaul of the Schengen area was reaffirmed by EU officers.[22] The Forum addressed five main topics regarding the Schengen area:

i operational and legislative changes to improve the area's monitoring and identification mechanisms;
ii revision of the SBC;
iii better management of EU's external borders, namely through the rapid implementation of the Entry/Exit System (EES) and of the European Traveller Information and Authorisation System (ETIAS), a visa waiver application process;

iv strengthening of police cooperation and information exchange; and
v strengthening of the Schengen area governance through Regular Schengen Forum meetings (European Commission, 2020j). In January 2021 the Commission launched a public consultation on the Future of the Schengen agreement.[23]

The pandemic crisis, as indeed other crises before it, opened a window of opportunity to resolve some long-identified problems affecting the Schengen area. At the time of writing the process of reform is underway. However, it is too soon to assess if this opportunity will turn into a lost one, as others did.

4.6 Conclusions

Freedom of movement is a building block of the EU. It is essential for the SM but it is also a crucial element of the European way of life. Although limitations to free movement, including internal border closures, were implemented on several occasions before the COVID-19 pandemic, the severity of the limitations adopted as a response to the current crisis was unprecedented. This raised questions regarding the necessity and the proportionality of the measures adopted. The chapter therefore tested the conformity of restrictions to free movement, particularly internal border controls, through the lens of European and international law. Ultimately, our goal was to understand the impact of these measures on the European integration process.

Our findings suggest that, from a procedural standpoint, member states generally complied. However, checked against the criteria that justifies an exception to free movement, member states' decisions do not exactly pass the test. Doubts remain as regards the necessity, proportionality and non-discrimination principles. That being said, member states' decisions were a normal reaction to an unknown threat. The securitisation of COVID-19 helped to legitimate exceptional measures, even if they severely limited citizens' rights. It is telling evidence that, at least during the first wave of the pandemics, those measures had the support of a large part of European citizens. Would this represent a fundamental shift in the way citizens perceive the importance of free movement? Although it is too soon for a definitive conclusion, the increasing contestation to new restrictions to movement during the second and third waves suggest that citizens' acceptance of the rules limiting their ability to move freely is circumstantial, resulting more from a sense of vulnerability and a belief that restrictions to movement were an important step to slow the spread of the virus than from a downgrading of the importance of free movement.

Border closure during the pandemic, and particularly the initial disarray of member states' decisions, brought to the surface old problems of the Schengen framework, opening the window of opportunity to reform. The Commission seized the opportunity and is committed to launch a Strategy on the Future of Schengen (early 2021) that could represent an overhaul of the Schengen framework. Again, the incremental reform seems to be the way forward.

Notes

1 The other three freedoms were related with goods, services and capital.
2 The Schengen area consists of 26 member countries, of which 22 are EU member states (Austria, Belgium, Czech Republic, Denmark, Estonia, Finland, France, Germany, Greece, Hungary, Italy, Latvia, Lithuania, Luxembourg, Malta, Netherlands, Poland, Portugal, Slovakia, Slovenia, Spain and Sweden), and four are non-EU member states with associate status (Iceland, Norway, Switzerland and Liechtenstein). See Schengen visa information. Available at: www.schengenvisainfo.com/schengen-visa-countries-list/ [Accessed 8 March 2021].
3 The sentence is in bold in the original.
4 The United Nations Secretary-General, António Guterres, Britain Prime-Minister Boris Johnson, or former US President Donald Trump are just a few examples. Interestingly enough, however, the de-securitisation strategy was also used by some political leaders, such as Brazilian President Jair Bolsonaro or Belarus's President Alexander Lukashenko, who have recurrently dismissed the threat (Vankovska, 2020, p. 73).
5 For example, a group of members of the World Emergency COVID-19 Pandemic Ethics (WeCope) Committee made an explicitly call to cease the use of war metaphors. See Arawi et al. (2020).
6 According to Kenwick and Simmons (2020, p. E41), 186 countries responded to COVID-19 with external border restrictions.
7 For a detailed overview of these rules see, for example, Carrera and Luk (2020, pp. 48–52).
8 See Directive 2004/38/EC of the European Parliament and of the Council of 29 April 2004 on the right of citizens of the Union and their family members to move and reside freely within the territory of the Member States amending Regulation (EEC) No 1612 /68 and repealing Directives 64/221/EEC, 68/360/EEC, 72/194/EEC, 73/148/EEC, 75/34/EEC, 75/35/EEC, 90/364/EEC, 90/365/EEC and 93/96/EEC. Available at: https://eur-lex.europa.eu/legal-content/EN/TXT/PDF/?uri=CELEX:32004L0038&from=en [Accessed 15 March 2021].
9 See for example SchengenVisaInf News. 'Only 11Member States Have Notified EU for Reintroduction of Internal Border Checks', 11 March 2020. Available at: www.schengenvisainfo.com/news/only-11-schengen-members-have-notified-eu-for-reintroduction-of-border-checks/ [Accessed 24 March 2021].
10 For a complete list of the notifications see Member States on the temporary reintroduction of border control at internal borders pursuant to Article 25 and 28 et seq. of the Schengen Borders Code. Available at: https://ec.europa.eu/home-affairs/sites/homeaffairs/files/what-we-do/policies/borders-and-visas/schengen/reintroduction-border-control/docs/ms_notifications_-_reintroduction_of_border_control.pdf [Accessed 24 March 2021].
11 ShengenVisaInformation.com. 'EU Commission Urges Six Member States to Remove Some of Their COVID-19 Border Restrictions', 24 February 2021. Available at: www.schengenvisainfo.com/news/eu-commission-urges-six-member-states-to-remove-some-of-their-covid-19-border-restrictions/ [Accessed 21 March 2021].

12 One example is the right to protest. For an analysis on how the pandemic response affected the right to protest see, for example, Narsee (2021).

13 Actually, the reference to the SM was recurrent in the Commission's documents related to mobility. Early in March 2020, when member states started to close internal borders, the Commission used the market (more specifically, the necessity to preserve the integrity of the SM) to establish common rules.

14 The Communication was part of a package of guidelines and recommendations related to tourism and transport to help member states gradually lift restrictions on free movement.

15 See European Council/Council of the European Union (2020) Video Conference of Home Affairs Ministers, 5 June 2020 Main Results. Available at: www.consilium.europa.eu/en/meetings/jha/2020/06/05/ [Accessed 19 March 2021].

16 The document included sections regarding test capacity, medical countermeasures, healthcare surge capacity, support to vulnerable groups, and seasonal influenza.

17 pplware.sapo. 'STAYAWAY COVID: 2,5 milhões de downloads! 4485 códigos gerados', 10 November 2020. Available at: https://pplware.sapo.pt/informacao/stayaway-covid-25-milhoes-de-downloads-4485-codigos-gerados/ [Accessed 24 March 2021].

18 The Recommendation was amended on 28 January 2021 in view of a very high level of community transmission across the EU, possibly linked to the increased transmissibility of the new SARS-CoV-2 variants. See Council of the European Union (2021) Council Recommendation amending Council Recommendation (EU) 2020/1475 of 13 October 2020 on a coordinated approach to the restriction of free movement in response to the COVID-19 pandemic, 5716/21. Available at: www.consilium.europa.eu/media/48122/st05716-en21-public.pdf [Accessed 21 March 2021].

19 See European Centre for Disease Prevention and Control. Maps in support of the Council Recommendation on a coordinated Approach to travel measures in the EU. Available at: www.ecdc.europa.eu/en/covid-19/situation-updates/weekly-maps-coordinated-restriction-free-movement [Accessed 19 March 2021].

20 Denmark, Bulgaria, Germany, Italy, France, Poland, Spain, Portugal and Sweden.

21 Germany, Netherlands, Denmark, Spain, France, Sweden, Italy and Belgium.

22 ETIAS News. 'EU Plans to Overhaul the Schengen Area", 2 December 2020. Available at: www.etiasvisa.com/etias-news/eu-overhaul-schengen-area [Accessed 24 March 2021].

23 Between 1 January and 16 March 2020 EU citizens, civil society and other stakeholders were invited to answer a ten questions questionnaire about their experiences with Schengen and the impact which the recent COVID-19 pandemic and long-lasting reintroductions of border checks at internal borders had on it. See European Commission Security & Border Management, New Schengen Strategy, Public Consultation. Available at: https://ec.europa.eu/info/law/better-regulation/have-your-say/initiatives/12838-Security-border-management-new-Schengen-strategy/public-consultation [Accessed 24 March 2021].

Bibliography

Amiel, S., 2021. Will COVID-19 Spark Reform of the EU's Borderless Schengen Area? *Euronews*, 3 March 2021. Available at: www.euronews.com/2021/03/02/will-covid-19-spark-reform-of-the-eu-s-borderless-schengen-area [Accessed 21 March 2021].

Arawi, T. et al., 2020. *A Call to Cease the Use of War Metaphors in the COVID-19 Pandemic*. Available at: www.researchgate.net/publication/342232798_A_Call_to_Cease_the_Use_of_War_Metaphors_in_the_COVID-19_pandemic [Accessed 15 March 2021].

Berrod, F. and Bruyas, P., 2020. European Union: Are Borders the Antidote to Covid-19 Pandemic? *The Conversation*, 17 April 2020. Available at: https://theconversation.com/european-union-are-borders-the-antidote-to-the-covid-19-pandemic-136643 [Accessed 9 March 2021].

Bossong, R., 2020. EU Border Security in a Time of Pandemic – Restoring the Schengen Regime in the Face of Old Conflicts and New Requirements for Public Health. *SWP Comment*, 28 June 2020. Available at: www.swp-berlin.org/10.18449/2020C28/ [Accessed 15 March 2021].

Buzan, B. and Hansen, L., 2009. *The Evolution of International Security Studies*. Cambridge: Cambridge University Press.

Buzan, B., Waever, O. and de Wilde, J., 1998. *Security: A New Framework for Analysis*. Boulder, CO: Lynne Rienner Publishers.

Carrera, S. and Luk, N. C., 2020. In the Name of COVID-19: Schengen Internal Border Controls and Travel Restrictions in the EU. *IPOL – Policy Department for Citizens' Rights and Constitutional Affairs*. Available at: www.europarl.europa.eu/thinktank/en/document.html?reference=IPOL_STU(2020)659506 [Accessed 15 March 2021].

Chetail, V., 2020. Crisis without Borders: What Does International Law Say About Border Closure in the Context of Covid-19? Frontiers in Political Science, 3 December 2020. https://doi.org/10.3389/fpos.2020.606307.

Chinazzi, M., Davis, J. T., Ajelli, M., Gioannini, C., Litvinova, M., Merler, S., Pastore y Piontti, A., Mu, K., Rossi, L., Sun, K., Viboud, C., Xiong, X., Yu, H., Halloran, M. E., Longini Jr., I. M. and Vespignani, A., 2020. The Effect of Travel Restrictions on the Spread of the 2019 Novel Coronavirus (COVID-19) outbreak. *Science*, 368, pp. 395–400. Available at: https://science.sciencemag.org/content/sci/368/6489/395.full.pdf [Accessed 11 March 2021].

Council of the European Union, 2020b. Draft Council Recommendation on a coordinated approach to the restriction of free movement in response to the COVID-19 pandemic. Available at: https://data.consilium.europa.eu/doc/document/ST-11689-2020-REV-1/en/pdf [Accessed 19 March 2021].

Cuyvers, A., 2017. Free Movement of Persons in the EU. In: E. Ugirashebuja, J. E. Ruhangisa, T. Ottervanger and A. Cuyvers, eds. *East African Community Law: Institutional, Substantive and Comparative EU Aspects*. Leiden: Brill, pp. 354–64.

Deen, B. and Kruijver, K., 2020. Corona: EU's Existential Crisis: Why the Lack of Solidarity Threatens Not Only the Union's Health and Economy, But Also Its Security. *Clingendael Alert*, April 2020. Available at: www.clingendael.org/sites/default/files/2020-04/Alert_Corona_Existential_Crisis_April_2020.pdf [Accessed 11 January 2021].

Dumbrava, C., 2020. Towards a Common EU Approach to Lifting Coronavirus-Related Restrictions on Freedom of Movement. *European Parliamentary Research Service, Briefing*, November 2020. Available at: www.europarl.europa.eu/thinktank/en/document.html?reference=EPRS_BRI(2020)659368 [Accessed 15 March 2021].

Erzen, B., Weber, M., and Sacchetti, S., 2020. Expert Voice: How COVID-19 Is Changing Border Control. *ICMPD – International Centre for Migration Policy*

Development. Available at: www.icmpd.org/news-centre/news-detail/expert-voice-how-covid-19-is-changing-border-control/ [Accessed 21 March 2021].

European Commission, 2017. Proposal for a Regulation of the European Parliament and of the Council amending Regulation (EU) 2016/399 as regards the rules applicable to the temporary reintroduction of border control at internal borders. COM(2017) 571 final. Available at: www.europarl.europa.eu/RegData/docs_autres_institutions/commission_europeenne/com/2017/0571/COM_COM(2017)0571_EN.pdf [Accessed 24 March 2021].

European Commission, 2020a. *Europe's Moment: Repair and Prepare for the Next Generation*. COM(2020) 456 final. Available at: https://eur-lex.europa.eu/legal-content/EN/TXT/PDF/?uri=CELEX:52020DC0456&from=EN [Accessed 24 November 2020].

European Commission, 2020b. Tackling COVID-19 disinformation: Getting the facts right. COM(2020) 8 final, 10 June 2020. Available at: https://eur-lex.europa.eu/legal-content/EN/TXT/PDF/?uri=CELEX:52020JC0008&from=EN. [Accessed 4 December 2020].

European Commission, 2020c. *Short-term EU health preparedness for COVID-19 outbreaks*. COM(2020) 318 final, 15 July 2020. Available at: https://eur-lex.europa.eu/resource.html?uri=cellar:f6fbab84-c749-11ea-adf7-01aa75ed71a1.0002.02/DOC_1&format=PDF. [Accessed 28 November 2020].

European Commission, 2020d. *Building a European Health Union: Reinforcing the EU's Resilience for Cross-Border Health Threats*. COM(2020) 724 final, 11 November 2020. Available at: https://eur-lex.europa.eu/legal-content/EN/TXT/PDF/?uri=CELEX:52020DC0724&from=EN. [Accessed 28 November 2020].

European Commission, 2020e. Commission Recommendation (EU) 2020/518, 8 April 2020 on a common Union toolbox for the use of technology and data to combat and exit from COVID-19 crisis, in particular concerning mobile applications and the use of anonymised mobility data. Available at: <https://eur-lex.europa.eu/legal-content/EN/TXT/PDF/?uri=CELEX:32020H0518&from=EN> [Accessed 24 March 2021].

European Commission, 2020f. Short-term EU health preparedness for COVID-19 outbreaks. COM(2020) 318 final, 15 July 2020. Available at: https://eur-lex.europa.eu/resource.html?uri=cellar:f6fbab84-c749-11ea-adf7-01aa75ed71a1.0002.02/DOC_1&format=PDF [Accessed 10 February 2021].

European Commission, 2020g. Proposal for a Council Recommendation on a coordinated approach to the restriction of free movement in response to the COVID-19 pandemic. COM(2020) 449 final. Available at: https://data.consilium.europa.eu/doc/document/ST-10487-2020-INIT/en/pdf [Accessed 19 March 2021].

European Commission, 2020h. *On a New Pact on Migration and Asylum*. COM(2020) 609 final. Available at: https://eur-lex.europa.eu/resource.html?uri=cellar:85ff8b4f-ff13-11ea-b44f-01aa75ed71a1.0002.02/DOC_3&format=PDF [Accessed 24 March 2021].

European Commission, 2020i. *Commission Work Programme 2021 A Union of Vitality in a World of Fragility*. COM(2020) 690 final. Available at: https://ec.europa.eu/info/sites/info/files/2021_commission_work_programme_en.pdf [Accessed 24 March 2021].

European Commission, 2020j. *European Commission Press Release First Schengen Forum: Towards a stronger and more resilient Schengen*. 30 November 2020.

Available at: https://ec.europa.eu/commission/presscorner/detail/en/ip_20_2232 [Accessed 24 March 2021].

European Commission, 2021. Proposal for a Regulation of the European Parliament and of the Council on a framework for the issuance, verification and acceptance of interoperable certificates on vaccination, testing and recovery to facilitate free movement during the COVID-19 pandemic (Digital Green Certificate). COM(2021) 130 final. Available at: https://ec.europa.eu/info/sites/info/files/en_green_certif_just_reg130_final.pdf [Accessed 20 March 2021].

European Council, 2020. Special meeting of the European Council (17, 18, 19, 20 and 21 July) – Conclusions. Available at: www.consilium.europa.eu/media/45109/210720-euco-final-conclusions-en.pdf [Accessed 21 March 2021].

European Parliament, 2020. European Parliament resolution of 19 June 2020 on the situation in the Schengen area following the COVID-19 outbreak (2020/2640(RSP)). Available at: www.europarl.europa.eu/doceo/document/TA-9-2020-0175_EN.pdf [Accessed 21 March 2021].

Ferhani, A. and Rushton, S., 2020. The International Health Regulations, COVID-19, and Bordering Practices: Who Gets In, What Gets Out and Who Gets Rescued? *Contemporary Security Policy*, 41(3), pp. 458–77.

Flusberg, S. J., Matlock, T. and Thibodeau, P. H., 2018. War Metaphors in Public Discourse. *Metaphor and Symbol,* 33(1), pp. 1–18. Available at: www.researchgate.net/publication/322238852_War_metaphors_in_public_discourse [Accessed 15 January 2021].

Grépin, K. A., Ho, T. L., Liu, Z., Summer, M., Piper, J., Worsnop, C. Z. and Kelley, L., 2020. Evidence of the Effectiveness of Travel-Related Measures During the Early Phase of the Covid-19 Pandemic: A Rapid Systematic Review. *MedRxiv*, doi: https://doi.org/10.1101/2020.11.23.20236703. Available at: www.medrxiv.org/content/10.1101/2020.11.23.20236703v1.full-text [Accessed 10 March 2021].

Hernández-Quevedo, C., Scarpetti, G., Webb, E., Shuftan, N., Williams, G. A., Birk, H. O., Jervelund, S. S., Krasnik, A. and Vrangbaek, K., 2020. Effective Contact Tracing and the Role of Apps: Lessons from Europe. *Eurohealth* 2020, 26(2), pp. 40–4. Available at: https://apps.who.int/iris/bitstream/handle/10665/336294/Eurohealth-26-2-40-44-eng.pdf [Accessed 24 March 2021].

Human Rights Watch, 2020. *Human Rights Dimensions of COVID-19 Response.* Available at: www.hrw.org/news/2020/03/19/human-rights-dimensions-covid-19-response# [Accessed 5 March 2021].

International Monetary Fund, 2020. *Policy Responses to COVID-19.* Available at: www.imf.org/en/Topics/imf-and-covid19/Policy-Responses-to-COVID-19#top. [Accessed 28 November 2020].

Kenwick, M. R. and Simmons, B. A., 2020. Pandemic Response as Border Politics. *International Organization*, 74(Supplement), pp. E36–E58.

Koikkalainen, S., 2011. Free Movement in Europe: Past and Present. *Migration Policy Institute.* Available at: www.migrationpolicy.org/article/free-movement-europe-past-and-present [Accessed 8 March 2021].

Kostakopoulou, D., 2013. *Co-creating European citizenship Policy Review.* European Commission, Directorate-General for Research & Innovation. Available at: https://gppq.fct.pt/brochuras/7pq/ssh/co-creating_eu_citizenship.pdf [Accessed 8 March 2021].

Lang, G., 2021. "Laws of Fear" in the EU: The Precautionary Principle and Public Health Restrictions to Free Movement of Persons in the Time of COVID-19.

European Journal of Risk Regulation, pp. 1–24. Available at: www.cambridge.org/core/journals/european-journal-of-risk-regulation/article/laws-of-fear-in-the-eu-the-precautionary-principle-and-public-health-restrictions-to-free-movement-of-persons-in-the-time-of-covid19/56741AF86D63D0465EC1AA364CA136CB [Accessed 5 March 2021].

Liu, X. and Bennett, M. M., 2020. Viral Borders: COVID-19's Effects on Securitization, Surveillance, and Identity in Mainland China and Hong Kong. *Dialogues in Human Geography*, 10(2), pp. 158–63.

Looi, M. K., 2020. Covid-19: Is a Second Wave Hitting Europe? *BJM 2020*, 371:m4113. Available at: www.bmj.com/content/bmj/371/bmj.m4113.full.pdf [Accessed 21 March 2021].

Marzocchi, O., 2020. *Free Movement of Persons. European Parliament Fact Sheets on the European Union*. Available at: www.europarl.europa.eu/ftu/pdf/en/FTU_4.1.3.pdf [Accessed 5 March 2021].

Montaldo, S., 2020. The COVID-19 emergency and the reintroduction of internal border controls in the Schengen area: Never let a serious crisis go to waste. Available at: www.europeanpapers.eu/en/system/files/pdf_version/EP_EF_2020_I_016_Stefano_Montaldo_00353.pdf [Accessed 5 March 2021].

Mortera-Martinez, C., 2020. Will the Coronavirus Pandemic Deliver a Coup de Grâce to Schengen? *Centre for European Reform*, 30 September 2020. Available at: www.cer.eu/publications/archive/bulletin-article/2020/will-coronavirus-pandemic-deliver-coup-de-grâce-schengen [Accessed 24 March 2021].

Murphy, M. P. A., 2021. The Double Articulation of Sovereign Bordering: Spaces of Exception, Sovereign Vulnerability, and Agamben's Schmitt/Foucault Synthesis. *Journal of Borderland Studies*, 36(4), pp. 599–615. https://doi.org/10.1080/08865655.2019.1683053.

Narsee, A., 2021. Europeans' Right to Protest Under Threat. *Carnegie Europe*, 27 January 2021. Available at: https://carnegieeurope.eu/2021/01/27/europeans-right-to-protest-under-threat-pub-83735 [Accessed 17 March 2021].

Petrequin, S., 2020. EU Countries Adopt Common Travel Guidelines amid Pandemic. *Associated Press News*, 13 October 2020. Available at: https://apnews.com/article/virus-outbreak-travel-international-news-business-pandemics-ceac3bbe3f024b4b96c54b172f849e20 [Accessed 19 March 2021].

Ramji-Nogales, J. and Lang, I. G., 2020. Freedom of Movement, Migration and Borders. *Journal of Human Rights*, 19(5), pp. 593–602.

Ramón, C., 2020. Opinion: 'Pandemicization': The New 'Securitization' in Cross Border and Travel Governance? *Bipartisan Policy Center*, 1 May 2020. Available at: https://bipartisanpolicy.org/blog/opinion-pandemicization-the-new-securitization-in-cross-border-and-travel-governance/ [Accessed 10 March 2021].

Sabat, I., Neuman-Bhome, S., Varghese, N. E., Barros, P. P, Brouwer, W., van Exel, J., Schreyogg, J. and Stargardt, T., 2020. United but Divided: Policy Responses and People's Perceptions in the EU during the COVID-19 Outbreak. *Health Policy*, 124, pp. 909–18.

Sánchez, S. I., 2015. Free Movement Law within the European Union: Workers, Citizens, and Third-Country Nationals. In: M. Panizzon, G. Zurcher and E. Fornalé, eds. *The Palgrave Handbook of International Labour Migration: Law and Policy Perspectives*. Basingstoke: Palgrave, pp. 361–81.

Semino, E., 2021. “Not Soldiers but Fire-Fighters” – Metaphors and Covid-19. *Health Communication*, 36(1), pp. 50–8. Available at: www.tandfonline.com/doi/epub/10.1080/10410236.2020.1844989?needAccess=true [Accessed 15 March 2021].

Silver, L., Fagan, M. and Kent, N. O., 2020. Majorities in the European Union Have Favourable Views of the Bloc. *Pew Research Center*. Available at: www.pewresearch.org/global/2020/11/17/majorities-in-the-european-union-have-favorable-views-of-the-bloc/ [Accessed 17 March 2021].

The Economist, 2020. Coronavirus Second Wave Hits Europe in Force. *Economist Intelligence Unit*, 3 November 2020. Available at: www.eiu.com/n/coronavirus-second-wave-hits-europe-in-force/ [Accessed 17 March 2021].

Vankovska, B., 2020. Dealing with COVID-19 in the European Periphery: Between Securitization and ‘Glaslighting’. *Journal of Global Faultlines*, 7(1), pp. 71–88.

Von der Leyen, U. and Michel, C., 2020. *Joint European Roadmap Towards Lifting COVID-19 Containment Measures*. 15 April 2020. Available at: https://op.europa.eu/en/publication-detail/-/publication/14188cd6-809f-11ea-bf12-01aa75ed71a1/language-en [Accessed 8 February 2021].

Zanin, M., and Papo, D., 2020. Travel Restrictions during Pandemics: A Useful Strategy? *Chaos 30*, 111103 (2020). Available at: https://aip.scitation.org/doi/pdf/10.1063/5.0028091 [Accessed 12 March 2021].

Zerka, P., 2020. Why Voters Support Both Stricter Borders and Respect for Human Rights. *ECFR*, 21 August 2020. Available at: https://ecfr.eu/article/commentary_why_voters_support_both_stricter_borders_and_respect_for_human_r/ [Accessed 17 March 2021].

5 Humanitarian emergency and the European Union

Solidarity, leadership and national reassurance

5.1 Introduction

This chapter deals with humanitarian emergency in the EU following the outbreak of COVID-19 and how emergency was coped with by relevant actors. The seriousness of the outbreak asked for contingency plans to mitigate the number of victims and the threat of contagion. At the outset, the initiative (and political leadership) belonged to national authorities. Paradoxically, a problem that affected all member states was not addressed through joint action. This conflicts with the rationale of joint action, which is distinctive of European integration. The exceptionality of the pandemic crisis was the input for the analysis that disturbed the regular functioning of the EU. The discussion of the chapter revolves around the consequences for European integration from the peculiarities of crisis management: was the inward, selfish position of national authorities consistent with the idiosyncrasy of European integration?

Section 5.2 addresses the chronology of events in the early surge of national political leadership (and inward-looking problem-solving as well), which dictated national reassurance beforehand, precluding the political initiative and the functioning of the decision-making process of the EU. Section 5.3 looks at the stage of inter-state solidarity when, finally, political willingness to act at the EU level emerged and the EU articulated with national authorities. An important case study underlying the prominence of the EU is the EU-wide programme of vaccination, which is the focus of Section 5.4. Section 5.5 turns into the normative dimension of the events encompassed in the chapter, discussing the impact of the overall reaction to the pandemic crisis to European integration, notably on what concerns the sanitary dimension. So far, how has the EU been muddling through the waters of the pandemic? Did the early period of national leadership and absent cooperation damage the EU?

5.2 Political reaction at the outset of the pandemic: national leadership and reassurance

The first signs of COVID-19 in European countries shed light on how unprepared political authorities were to handle the sanitary crisis. The

DOI: 10.4324/9781003153900-6

huge contagious potential and how the virus was quickly progressing in all European countries led to a self-centred reaction. Each country was on its own, trying to contain the contagious effects of the disease as much as it was possible (Alemanno, 2020). During the early stage (early March to mid-May 2020), a paradoxical effect was undistinguishable of the disarray that affected countries: since the sanitary crisis was hitting all countries and, thus, the crisis was symmetric in nature, all conditions were ideal for joint crisis management. Yet, instead of promoting cooperation, or allowing (at the level of the EU) supranational institutions to play a role in the strategy to deal with the crisis, national authorities promoted unilateral solutions and refused to adopt a joint decision-making process aiming at mitigating the early effects of COVID-19. Panic might explain how bewildered national authorities were (Roberto, Johnson and Rauhaus, 2020). In their understanding, national interests prevailed. Isolation was, therefore, the first card in their hand as they had to provide solutions to a disease that, nevertheless, was not entirely unknown.

What is puzzling in the early weeks of the political reaction to the spread of COVID-19 is that national authorities were not caught by surprise. The virus flew from the East to the West. At the outset (late 2019, early 2020), the virus affected the Asian countries. The prospect of a pandemic was real, as experts warned that sooner or later, the West would also become under the spell of the pandemic (Nicola et al., 2020) (see also Chapter 2). It was just a matter of time before European countries were knocked out by the sanitary crisis. Instead of a proactive strategy that collected valuable information on the experience of Asian countries affected by the virus, national authorities in Europe seemed to be dormant. In this context, inaction (or, to put it better, the absence of a proactive stance) was a negative surprise.

It seems that national authorities misjudged the lethality of the pandemic and neglected the dramatic contagious potential of the virus. With the benefit of hindsight, at the time of writing (April 2021), the idea that a preventive strategy was ruled out comes to the surface. Inertia is hardly understandable, as the knowledge of the intimidating effects of the sanitary crisis in Asian countries was already at the disposal of experts and politicians. EU institutions lagged behind, since they missed the opportunity to put the issue at the forefront of political concerns and to draw the attention of national governments. Yet, their inertia is mostly explained by the fact that national authorities' hyper-activism followed apathy, thereby suffocating the visibility of the action of EU institutions (Fetzer et al., 2020).

The cost of neglecting prevention was hysteria when, finally, European countries were also under the radar of COVID-19. It seems that political authorities were waiting for the virus to arrive to design a strategy to contain its progression. Decisions at the beginning were not different from countries that were previously affected by the disease. Instead of capitalising on the knowledge of countries affected in the first place, European countries only reacted when the sanitary crisis unveiled. They squandered the knowledge spread after Asian countries' early experience with COVID-19. In addition, national governments decided to promote ad-hoc, non-cooperative solutions, as if each country had problems on its own (Anderson, Mckee and Mossialos, 2020). They were acting as if the pandemic did not exist. As a pandemic, the symptoms of the disease are the same irrespective of the country affected by it. It is a symmetric crisis. All countries are affected, one way or the other. Considering the symmetric nature of the COVID-19 pandemic, it is difficult to understand why national governments decided to act on their own, as if the problem was only affecting each country and not all other countries – as if the effects, both at the sanitary level and at many other dimensions, were not roughly the same from country to country (Moreira and Hick, 2021).

At the same time, the virus did not stop at national borders. This makes it particularly difficult to understand why national governments decided to close borders when the disease was already spread all over Europe. On politicians' judgements, the awareness of how interconnected regions, countries and continents are was left behind. Travelling facilities are a key feature of contemporary globalisation. It is increasingly easy to fly from one country to another, even when formal border controls are still taking place (which is not the case of EU member states that ratified the Schengen Agreement). These aspects, together with the nature of the virus (notably, the huge potential of contagion), should have motivated national governments (and the EU, as well) to try to anticipate the consequences of the pandemic. While the virus was spreading and killing people in Asian countries, no European country decided to raise travel restrictions (or even a travel ban, as it was commonplace at a later stage) or to administer viral tests to persons coming from countries affected by the virus. The Commission was discrete. It could have warned national governments to undertake preventive measures to stop the propagation of the virus. To this extent, national authorities but also the Commission are not exempted from criticisms for their negligible approach to the sanitary crisis (Uddin et al., 2020).

Disarray is not the appropriate context for reasonable solutions. Considering the devastating potential of the pandemic owing to high ratios of transmissibility of the virus, national governments were prompt to decide on a lockdown. This political decision was guided by two imperatives: (i) a sanitary imperative – to prevent the propagation of the virus by sending the maximum number of people home. It was expected that isolation at home would put a break on the chain of the contagion. This was the precondition to curb down the pervasive effects of the disease (Karnon, 2020); and (ii) a humanitarian imperative – the impact of the virus was irregular on persons, as some were severely affected (notably older persons and those who were already exposed to other pathologies) while others remained asymptomatic when contaminated by the virus, which further raised the prospect of contagion. Lockdown was also responsive to humanitarian conditions since it was pivotal to save human lives (Balmford et al., 2020).

In addition to lockdown, restrictions on the mobility of persons were imposed. Only when countries were hit by an increasing number of positive cases the death toll started to rise, and anxiety and difficulties with the healthcare system were escalating, national authorities decided to put a break on the mobility of citizens coming from other countries (Gatto et al., 2020). In extreme cases, local sanitary fences were raised, so that mobility from town to town or from village to village was prohibited (Bonardi et al., 2020). These measures were decided at the national level without enlisting cooperation with other countries (in some cases, the decision to close borders was approved by the authorities of the countries with shared borders) or by promoting cooperation at the EU level. Each country was acting on its own, as if the EU did not exist and the pandemic was not a pandemic with the embedded symmetric effects.

Since the crisis was, first and foremost, a sanitary crisis, the dimension concerning public health was on the top of national governments' priorities. Massive resources were allocated to hospitals so that they could adjust to the increasing inflow of patients suffering from COVID-19 (Bénassy-Quéré et al., 2020). The provision of basic materials to treat patients ranked high in governments' priorities. This was particularly important for ventilators, as patients in worse health condition needed intubation and constant monitoring by ventilators (Goniewicz et al., 2020). At some point, resources available were not enough to meet the necessities owing to the large increase in the number of infected persons who were on hospital beds in a serious condition. The response at the beginning was strictly national, with no articulation between national authorities. One dramatic episode going back to the early stage of the outbreak reminds of the Italian government's plea for other EU member states to receive some patients due to overcrowded hospitals. The evidence of national strict self-centredness was the absence of reaction of other national governments. They were unwilling to receive Italian patients as they were affected by the uncertain evolution of the pandemic in their own countries.[1] Each country was left on their own as a consequence of a non-coordinated action. Later, Ursula von der Leyen recognised how shameful this episode was, and she apologised in the name of the Commission for the inaction to the Italian government's request.[2]

EU institutions also came under national authorities' criticism concerning the lack of a proactive stance. Maybe it was time for EU institutions to take the initiative and, at least, try to raise national governments' awareness of the severity of the sanitary crisis that lay ahead. If national governments remained unresponsive, EU institutions (notably those that are free from the input of national governments: the Commission and the EP) could play a proactive role and move ahead by warning societies at large about the pandemic that was getting closer to Europe.

Perhaps the prudence of the Commission owes, to a large extent, to the fact that it was recently appointed (1 December 2019). A recently appointed institution that pleads political attention has weak political conditions to come to the limelight and promote the political initiative of waking up national governments to the seriousness of the sanitary crisis that was knocking at the door of European countries. In addition, the appointment of the new Commission was surrounded by controversy. The *spitzankandidaten* procedure (enacted by the Lisbon Treaty and implemented to the appointment of the previous Commission headed by Jean-Claude Juncker) was not followed, which led to criticisms about the democratic legitimacy of the Commission and affected the political visibility of the institution when it came into office (Müller Gómez and Thieme, 2020).

5.3 Time for solidarity and joint action: the European Union comes into the fore

After a period of chaos and dismay where the pandemic was addressed at the national level, member states realised that the nature of the problem required a different approach. The political reaction at the outset had, at least, the potential to break the accelerated increase of the number of infected persons. The outbreak of COVID-19 was contained after two months of strict lockdown in EU member states,[3] as statistical data finally showed a downward evolution (Sheikh et al., 2020). Yet, the authorities were aware that the fight against the sanitary crisis was not over, as experts warned that a second wave was expected to start in the autumn (Middleton et al., 2020). In addition to the non-sanitary aspects of the crisis (explored in other chapters of the book), pure public health considerations did not vanish from the political landscape.

The awareness of how an ongoing strategy was necessary, which in turn required adjustments as the process developed, made national governments realise that it was time for cooperation and to articulate in the context of the EU. Amidst the grimness of the situation, it was time to settle down and to reassess the rationale of the early reaction to the pandemic. The Commission finally gained ground, as it came up as the coordinator of national efforts to tackle the negative implications of COVID-19 (Wolff and Ladi, 2020) (see also Chapter 2 for a detailed background of how the Commission emerged as an actor of crisis management). Member states' evolution was monitored by the Commission. The institution acted as a *locus* for the gathering of important information concerning the spread of the disease and member states' strategies (Pacces and Weimer, 2020). At the same time, national ministers agreed to coordinate their efforts in the Council and in the European Council, bringing the supranational level to the forefront. Ministers of Health engaged in the Council, articulating the expertise to lay down a strategy to mitigate the effects of the sanitary crisis (Brooks, de Ruijter and Greer, 2021). Coordination of efforts between national governments through the mediation of the EU institution where they have a seat showed a different methodology to address the pandemic. Cooperation and interaction finally ranked high in member states' perception of the crisis. The rationale of common problems addressed through a strategy that emphasised joint action took hold and national politicians started to talk with each other. Finally, crisis management was focused on the supranational level.

At the same time, openness of member states to other countries' necessities meant that national governments ended the self-centred approach to the pandemic crisis, and that inter-state solidarity was taking place. That happened for the first time in late March 2020, when German hospitals received Italian and French patients due to excessive capacity in these countries' hospitals.[4]

It is difficult to find an answer on whether the emergency of the EU was the outcome of national governments' awareness that the EU was the appropriate decision-making arena for going against the sanitary crisis, or just the outcome of national level's awareness that the most dramatic stage of the pandemic was left behind. The distinction of scenarios is not meaningless, as it entails important consequences for the position of the EU in the context of the pandemic crisis (as Section 5.4 will explore). Signs coming from politicians' statements are, nevertheless, unclear (Van Schaik, Jørgensen and van de Pas, 2020).

On the one hand, the unambiguous introduction of the EU in the range of actors dealing with COVID-19 happened when the number of cases was slowing down. The reasonable explanation is that national governments gave the floor to the EU when the pandemic was not so dramatic, despite all signs of uncertainty that public health experts and epidemiologists were constantly voicing. If this interpretation holds, the impression is that the national level was given priority to tackle the most dramatic stage of the sanitary crisis, while the EU played a role when the goal was to control the evolution of the pandemic. The national level monopolised the stage when the problems were more intense, and the supranational level was asked to step in when mitigating the sanitary crisis was at stake. Accordingly, an imbalance between national governments and the EU is implied in this reading of the events. The focus on the national level reveals the perceived self-reliance of member states when they were struck by the uncontrolled development of COVID-19. They acted as if the purest rationale of supranational integration did not apply to a joint problem with the dimension of a pandemic. Maybe this portrays the nature of European integration sealed throughout the history of the EU: in times of intense crisis, national governments take the centre stage and downplay the intervention of the EU, thereby decreasing the status of the EU as a polity (Bouckaert et al., 2020).

What is interesting is that at the early stage of the pandemic crisis in the European continent the number of persons infected by COVID-19 and the death toll were not at its peak, as the second wave (from autumn 2020 onwards) (Coccia, 2020) and the third wave (early 2021 onwards)[5] showed a statistical increase in both the number of dead persons and the number of persons infected by the virus. Yet, at this time the reaction to the revival of COVID-19 was not national governments' exclusive prerogative, as they seem to have realised the benefits of pooling their efforts in the institutional system of the EU (Greer, Ruijter and Brooks, 2020). This is an interesting finding since the second and, especially, the third waves of COVID-19 seem more extensive and resilient to counteractive measures (which includes the beginning of vaccination) than it was the first wave.

A possible explanation pegs to the learning effects of the virus and the human reaction to it. In the early stages of the pandemic, actors were caught by surprise (if the expression is acceptable, considering that learning was available through the implications of the sanitary crisis in Asian countries) and they were therefore dominated by panic, dismissing cooperation with other countries and the intervention of the EU. Almost one year after the outbreak of the sanitary crisis in Europe, experts and decision-makers learned about the virus; policymakers at least learned, with the support of scientific expertise, the appropriate measures to prevent the spread of the disease. The sense of urgency (and disarray) was not so forceful as it was in the early days of the pandemic. National governments were aware of the idiosyncrasies of the virus and recognised the need of joint action and solidarity as the building blocks for efficient crisis management.

On the other hand, unclear prospects about the evolution of the pandemic shed light on the likelihood that the number of cases would increase again with foreseeable new waves and strains of the virus. This reinforced the perception that joint action at the level of the EU was required. At the same time, it sends opposite signals about the relevance of the EU. A sound strategy was designed when the anomalous status of the pandemic was washed away, as experts pointed out for the expected resilience of the virus and its long-term effects together with the learning effects coming from previous months that inspired a certain sense of 'normality' going back to societies (Oswick, Grant and Oswick, 2020). National governments were not prominent as before and leverage to coordination of efforts in the context of the EU was recognised.

An obstacle prevented a comprehensive intervention of the EU: according to the constitutional settlement of the EU, the national level is endowed with the large bulk of competences on the healthcare system and the design of public health policy. At best, the EU enjoys powers of support in this policy area, which leaves the design of healthcare systems and the most important decisions concerning the functioning of public health policy in the hands of national governments (Hervey and Vanhercke, 2010). Since the crisis was first and foremost a sanitary crisis, crisis management outlined public health policy measures (Bargain and Aminjonov, 2020). Hence, the emphasis on national decision-making. Still, each national government was not left to its own, as they perceived the need to interact for their countries were affected by a symmetric crisis. This perception gave a role to the EU, yet a role that is not comparable with the one played by national governments when it comes to taking commensurate decisions requiring policy design.

Throughout the crisis, an imbalance between member states and the EU (when viewed from the perspective of different polities) was striking. Clearly, national governments were the centripetal actor, while the EU was given a secondary role. This is not to say that the role of EU institutions was negligible. At one level, the Commission did its job as a policy entrepreneur, as the President of the Commission, Ursula von der Leyen, did not hesitate in positioning herself as a high-profile actor in the ongoing management of the pandemic crisis (Emiliani, 2020). Additionally, national governments acknowledged how useful the institutional system of the EU is to coordinate national efforts and to extract learning effects from member states that were considered as successful cases of accommodation to the challenges of the pandemic crisis (Aubrecht et al., 2020). This recognition reinforced the role of the EU in the contingency plan to COVID-19.

Notwithstanding more was expected from the EU, since the pandemic was a symmetric crisis and the rationale of joint problem-solving was innate to the sanitary crisis, the costs of contextualisation (when countries first became affected by COVID-19 cases and disarray and non-cooperative solutions emerged) explain the constraints on EU action. The strategy of vaccination, indeed, an EU-wide strategy, was the turning point on how humanitarian emergency was shaped in the EU.

5.4 The EU-wide programme of vaccination

As the intensity of COVID-19 waned, and the number of persons infected and the death toll decreased, the positive effects of lockdown became clear (but not unanimously, as some authors were critical of the damages to individual rights that restrictions tied to lockdown implied; see Chapter 6). At the same time, the devastation on the economy was outstanding (as Chapter 3 explored). A difficult balance between controlling COVID-19 and allowing the proper functioning of the economy was at stake since the beginning of the sanitary crisis. A trade-off between saving lives at the cost of the economy or preserving the economy at the expense of human lives was the underlying challenge. Yet, as the pandemic started to push backwards, the pendulum swung towards the economy (Favero, Ichino and Rustichini, 2020).

At the same time, it was time to breathe fresh air after the dramatic weeks of the beginning of the pandemic. Aside from negotiations about economic recovery that were taking place at the level of the EU (see Chapter 3), contingency in the sanitary dimension was still alive. According to experts, the downward spiral of COVID-19 just meant that radical lockdown gave an input to mitigate the penetration of the virus. Nonetheless, the virus thrived and the potential of a contagion, and hence of fuelling the pandemic again, was still a threat pending over societies (and decision-makers, in particular). Experts stressed that vaccines were the only prescription to defeat the virus and to restore some sense of 'normality' to societies (Veugelers and Zachmann, 2020). In addition, since restrictions were lifted for the sake of economy, the combination of a society freed from lockdown with the wonders of summertime and the timing necessary to prepare vaccines was indicative that a second wave was very likely to take place somewhere in the autumn of 2020. Vaccines are a precondition to tear down COVID-19 but also to mitigate the expected effects of the second and (possibly, at that time) the third wave of the pandemic.

The decision to order the COVID-19 vaccines jointly contributed to reinforce the image of Union. On 17 June 2020, the Commission unveiled an EU vaccine strategy based on two pillars: '[s]ecuring sufficient production of vaccines and thereby sufficient supplies for its Member States' and '[a]dapting the EU's regulatory framework to the current urgency' (European Commission, 2020, p. 2). In the Strategy, the Commission made it clear that individual action would only lead to suboptimal results:

> [j]oint action at EU level is the surest, quickest and most efficient way of achieving that objective. No Member State on its own has the capacity to secure the investment in developing and producing a sufficient number of vaccines. A common strategy allows better hedging of bets, sharing of risks and pooling investments to achieve economies of scale, scope and speed.
>
> (European Commission, 2020, pp. 2–3)

The idea that joint procurement would avoid competition between member states was also explicitly stressed by the Commission (European Commission, 2020, p. 3). To that end, the Commission negotiated and concluded agreements with sixth[6] pharmaceutical companies to purchase COVID-19 vaccines. The first contract the Commission has negotiated on behalf of member states with a pharmaceutical company (AstraZeneca) entered into force on 27 August 2021. The Strategy was followed by several Commission communications on accelerating the preparedness for COVID-19 member states' vaccination strategies, vaccine deployment and on additional COVID-19 response measures (European Centre for Disease Prevention and Control, 2021b). To reaffirm the idea of unity, the Commission even suggested a common 'vaccine day' to initiate the vaccination campaign across the EU:

> [d]oses of the vaccine approved today will be available for all EU countries, at the same time, on the same conditions. The upcoming European vaccination days will also be a great moment of unity. This is a good way to end this difficult year, and to start turning the page on this pandemic. We are all in this together.
>
> (von der Leyen, 2020d)

A minor setback hampered the 'vaccine day', nevertheless. Three member states (Germany, Hungary and Slovakia) broke the gentleman's agreement between the Commission and national governments and started the vaccination one day ahead the planned date.[7] Interestingly, no controversy surrounded the decision of the three member states since criticisms were muted. These national governments were not accused of violating a duty of loyalty vis-à-vis other member states and the Commission. If anything, the episode is illustrative of how national egoism prevailed and how some national interests undo the commitment towards common interests even in times of emergency that affect all member states. Perhaps the episode did not give rise to critical voices considering the exceptional circumstances the EU was living in and the glimpse of hope embedded at the beginning of vaccination against COVID-19. It is our understanding that the desertion of Germany, Hungary and Slovakia did not hinder the central role played by the Commission during the transition from the critical period of the first wave of the pandemics to vaccination. The episode does not deserve a thorough analysis, not least it can be understood as an example of national reassurance. Indeed, these national governments' motivation existed. Nonetheless, it is located at the meso-level and, therefore, it does not thwart the centripetal role of the Commission.

Massive investment was injected into companies and research institutes where research for producing a vaccine against COVID-19 was taking place. According to the literature (Prudêncio and Costa, 2020), the amount of money invested in the research for these vaccines was unprecedented. Recent literature is consensual on recognising this is why vaccines were available in a short period of time, considering the requirements established by tight protocols and the several stages of experimentation that must be met before regulators accept the vaccine into the market (Kim, Dema and Reyes-Sandoval, 2020). Political pressure on pharmaceutical companies and laboratories mounted as well, as political authorities were aware of how crucial vaccines were for immunising the population against the effects of the virus (Iserson, 2021). According to some reports, the time between early research and the availability of vaccines was astonishing (Graham, 2020). Previous records have been broken. Since the problem was massive and life-threatening at a large scale, it is not surprising that efforts concentrated on research, experimentation and production of vaccines against COVID-19 were unprecedented. The means were of the similar scale of the problems affecting societies.

Despite the astonishing results that came from global scale mobilisation and collaboration of the scientific community, the industry was not immune to economic criteria and, what is more, the inevitable discrepancy between demand and supply of COVID-19 vaccines started to cause tensions and dissensions. When member states' vaccination campaign was expected to reach a steady pace, some pharmaceutical companies (such as AstraZeneca and BioNTech/Pfizer) announced that they would not be able to deliver the purchased doses of COVID-19 vaccines within the agreed timeframe. Companies justified the delays with manufacturing disruptions, resulting from shortages of important raw materials and other components in worldwide supply chains. As the EU appeared to be trailing behind the United Kingdom, the United States and Israel, the coronavirus vaccine 'blame game' (Deutsch, 2021) (re)appeared, with the Commission as the scapegoat (see Chapter 2). Accusations of unnecessary delays in vaccines' authorisation due to red tape, excessive concern on securing low process and underestimation of the doses needed, fuelled the debate.

The President of the Commission, in a speech before the EP, recognised the weaknesses of the EU's action:

> (…) the fact is that today we are not where we want to be in combating the virus. We were late in granting authorisation. We were too optimistic about mass production. And maybe we also took for granted that the doses ordered would actually arrive on time.
>
> (von der Leyen, 2021)

But also emphatically reaffirmed the advantages of joint procurement:

> (…) it was right – and is right – that we Europeans ordered our vaccine jointly and that we are now sharing it in a spirit of solidarity. I don't even want to imagine what it would have meant if some large Member States had secured the vaccine while the rest went empty-handed. What would that have meant for our internal market, and for European unity? It would have made no economic sense. And it would have meant the end of our Community.
>
> (von der Leyen, 2021)

Although some criticisms might be substantiated, at the time of writing it remains to be proved that a 'every man for himself' strategy would serve better the interests of EU citizens than concerted action.

Despite the unease resulting from the EU vaccination strategy hurdles, the fact remains that during the third wave (which hit the EU in late 2020 and early 2021), coordination between EU national governments became routine. When the growing number of persons infected and the rise of the death toll forced international organisations (notably the WHO), the EU and national governments paid attention to the revival of the pandemic. New strains of the virus (the British, the Brazilian, the South African, the Californian and the Indian) dictated its mutation, making COVID-19 prone to increased contagious potential and to infect youngsters. This changing pattern, in turn, threw new variables into the table that raised the concern of all actors involved in the fight against the sanitary crisis. Irrespective of the impressive records of new contaminations and patients killed by the virus all over Europe (and in other regions as well), national authorities did not promote an inward approach to the spread of COVID-19 and, instead, reinforced cooperation and joint decision.[8]

A good example is the 21 January 2021 meeting of the European Council. At this time, countries were severely affected by the third wave of the pandemic, albeit a mixed record was observed from country to country. Countries that restricted the circulation of persons during Christmas had less cases and deaths than countries that allowed some flexibility and made it possible for families to spent time together during Christmas.[9] If the latter were suffering the delayed consequences of an unwise decision (when viewed from the benefit of hindsight, one must recognise), even countries where a restricted policy was implemented were hit by the new wave of the pandemic. What is significant is all national governments' perception that the pandemic was a symmetric crisis (although some variation was noted on the number of positive cases per million of inhabitants) (Celi, Guarascio and Simonazzi, 2020) and, hence, the design of appropriate measures was tabled at the higher political level.

Crucially, as well, the 21 January 2021 European Council decided that borders should remain open, eliminating the prospect of closed borders (European Council/Council of the European Union, 2021) (as some press aired[10]). The decision to keep borders open is more than just a symbolic one. On the one hand, the actors involved avoided disarray despite the third wave of the pandemic raised alarm. On the other hand, the impression that a thoughtful decision was agreed is revealing of how actors incorporated the learning effects of the previous stages of the pandemic crisis. This was, to some extent, a message of confidence they conveyed to the public.

A few weeks later, nonetheless, a pandemic spike raised apprehension in some member states. Governments decided to impose restrictions on the circulation and implemented border controls.[11] At the time of writing (early April 2021), this is the instructive evidence of how uncertainty still prevails in the evolution of the pandemic, and to what extent political decisions still follow a volatile pattern. COVID-19 vagaries determine manifold 'unknown unknowns' (Grech, 2020).

5.5 Normative discussion: the reaction to COVID-19 and the development of the European Union

Two distinctive stages characterised the reaction to the pandemic. At the outset, the emphasis on decision-making at the national level superseded the supranational level. At a later stage (when decreasing incidence of COVID-19 followed severe lockdown and the closing of borders), the focus was gradually shifted towards the EU. Despite the analysis in this section being provisional (at the time of writing: early April 2021, when the severity of the third wave of the pandemic triggered the alarm among national authorities and EU institutions), our tentative findings start from the acknowledgement that a change of relevant actors took place in the due course of the adjustment to the pandemic, and whether this shift produced consequences for European integration.

An analysis of the early weeks of the pandemic might have been instructive of how the EU did not count. National reassurance was the key aspect that cut across all member states, leaving the EU outside. One might be tempted to avow that this was detrimental to the EU, maybe adding to the downgrading of European integration, especially when European countries were facing severe contingency. This is not our understanding. As emphasised earlier in this chapter (see Sections 5.2 and 5.3), national reassurance and the underlying denial of solidarity among member states was short-lived. In no circumstance the episode is revealing of how the EU was neglected, or even of the EU's diminished visibility in comparison with the intense (re)action of national authorities.

The exuberance of the national level signals how hysteria prevailed in national governments, not as an intentional action that downplayed the potential of the EU to address the pandemic crisis. Differently, if the early trend of national reassurance endured, with national governments' inward-looking stance preventing EU institutions from taking stock of the pandemic, a negative impact for European integration could be validated as one conspicuous implication of the pandemic crisis. This was not confirmed after the early stage of national authorities' overwhelming presence. As it was mentioned throughout this chapter, at some point the EU emerged at the decision-making level to address the sanitary crisis (in its plural dimensions) and national authorities also realised they should interact in the context of the institutional system of the EU.

Our understanding was confirmed with subsequent developments of the pandemic. Europe witnessed a second and a third waves of the pandemic and the EU was still in the driver's seat. Actors involved in addressing the pandemic crisis showed how they were sensitive to ongoing learning effects of the sanitary crisis, and albeit the number of infected persons and the death toll increased, especially during the third wave, they did not capitulate to a frenetic, although disordered, reaction to the acceleration of the disease. There was no evidence of national reassurance. This shows how the rationale changed and the challenge of humanitarian emergency required continuous joint action instead of each national government pulling disorderly in every direction. At the same time, the pandemic was an 'existential threat for the EU' (Wolff and Ladi, 2020, p. 1025).

The inter-temporal dynamics of adjustment to the pandemic crisis highlights how the EU emerged as a pivotal actor. This in turn, adds to the political visibility of the EU. Hence, COVID-19 triggered the actorness of the EU in the crisis management context that followed (Stahl, 2020). The circumstance is not a unique pattern in the history of European integration. Some literature points at the reaction to manifold crises, and how the European Communities/EU muddled through, as an instructive evidence of how European integration has developed in the aftermath of these crises (Schimmelfennig, 2017). It is not, however, the only input to the development of the EU, as other critical junctures played a role. It is important to recognise that: (i) the development of European integration is an outcome of both positive events (political willingness to make the EU move forward) and negative events (where different crises have played a role, acting as a push-in factor to expand the influence of the EU); (ii) following this trend, the adjustment to the pandemic crisis stands out as the corroboration of how the EU rises during a crisis and in its aftermath. Indeed,

> [a]fter initial responses that appeared to be a disappointing replay of previous crises, EU governance in the Covid-19 crisis may very well result in paradigmatic change toward deeper European integration in some areas, incremental change in others, or even reversal toward dis-integration in yet others (…) [showing a] more positive dynamics of interaction among EU actors during the pandemic, in contrast to the Eurozone.
>
> (Schmidt, 2020, p. 1177)

We argue that the stability of the role performed by the EU (especially the input of the Commission for the vaccination plan and the full range of political-economic measures approved to address the social and economic effects of COVID-19 explored in Chapter 3) is an evidence of how the sanitary crisis created the opportunity for the primacy of the EU in crisis management. We will not unveil an oracle, for social sciences are averse to a speculative educated guess. Yet, we wonder whether the learning effects of previous crises, to which the learning effects of the ongoing pandemic must be added, are the building blocks for reinforcing the EU as the appropriate locus for crisis management in the days to come in the face of other critical junctures. It is our understanding, at the time of writing, that the pandemic crisis made 'more Europe' possible.

5.6 Conclusions

The assessment of political actorness during the evolution of the pandemic crisis reveals how national authorities gave way to the EU in the context of crisis management triggered by humanitarian emergency. It is not a cynical insight, but it is fair to recognise that the pandemic promoted the reliance of (and on) the EU. After an early period of disorientation, in which national authorities denied cooperation and even joint decision for a problem that was affecting them all the same way, the EU became the optimal decision-making level to articulate a common strategy to hold up the propagation of COVID-19. From a normative standpoint, the shift of focus from the national to the supranational level equates to a strengthening of the EU.

Yet, the analysis cannot escape the proper context of European integration. The idiosyncrasy of the EU as a polity is at stake, especially how different decision-making layers interact (both within the institutional system of the EU and outside it, among and within national and sub-national authorities) to govern the EU, understood not only as the polity itself, but also member states. Notwithstanding the Commission promotes itself as a policy entrepreneur, decisions always require the cooperation between the EP and the Council of the EU. Developments that foster the role of the EU need the consent of national governments. Despite we acknowledging that 'more Europe' is one outcome of the way the pandemic crisis was addressed, an overstatement must be avoided. Indeed, the EU gained salience, but national governments accepted the coordination of efforts within the EU institutional system.

Outside the activism of the Commission (a rational undertaking, considering how this institution envisaged the crisis as a window of opportunity to trigger policy initiative) (Vesan, Corti and Sabato, 2021), the deepening of European integration tied to the management of the pandemic crisis was possible because member states promoted that role for the EU.

For this reason – let alone the early stage of disarray in which national governments ruled out interaction through the EU – it is an exaggeration to conclude that the EU was the winner. What is fair to recognise is that, once again, EU's increased visibility came alongside a critical background when the EU and member states were affected by an unprecedented pandemic. It is also reasonable to acknowledge that joint decision-making at the EU level provided efficient solutions to address COVID-19, although at some point (February 2021) difficulties in the provision of vaccines revealed the fragility of the Commission's strategy in the negotiations with pharmaceuticals. Yet, it is our understanding that this episode does show the fragility of the Commission (and the EU itself), but only reveals some naivety of the negotiation strategy devised. We do not follow the sceptical assessment of the Commission's role on the vaccination strategy (Verhofstadt, 2021).

To that extent, the role of the EU has not only to be recognised but also praised. It is a manifestation that in critical times, when a dauting prospect wrecks member states, it makes sense to act together through the institutional system of the EU instead of focusing on national, inward-looking solutions that expose national governments to paradoxical autarky. To prevent this paradox from taking place is precisely what European integration is mostly about.

Notes

1 *Financial Times*. "Italy Wonders Where Europe's Solidarity Is as Coronavirus Strains Show". 13 March 2020. Available online at: www.ft.com/content/d3bc25ea-652c-11ea-b3f3-fe4680ea68b5 [Accessed 18 January 2021].

2 BBC News. 'Coronavirus: EU Offers "Heartfelt Apology" to Italy". 16 April 2020. Available online at: www.bbc.com/news/world-europe-52311263 [Accessed 18 January 2021].

3 BBC News. 'Coronavirus: European Countries Further Relax Restrictions'. 18 May 2020. Available online at: www.bbc.com/news/world-europe-52701621 [Accessed 19 January 2021].

4 *Independent*. '"Solidarity Knows No Borders": Germany treating dozens of Coronavirus patients From Italy and France'. 1 April 2020. Available online at: www.independent.co.uk/news/world/europe/coronavirus-germany-italy-france-hospital-treatment-covid-19-a9440906.html [Accessed 19 January 2021].

5 EU Science Hub. 'COVID-19 Media Surveillance – 14 January 2021'. Available online at: https://ec.europa.eu/jrc/en/science-update/covid-19-media-surveillance-14-january-2021 [Accessed 18 January 2021].

6 BioNTech-Pfizer, Sanofy-GSK, Johnson & Johnson, CureVac, Moderna and AstraZeneca.

7 *The New York Times*. "Germany and Hungary Begin Vaccinations a Day Earlier'. 26 December 2020. Available online at: www.nytimes.com/2020/12/26/world/Germany-Hungary-vaccinations-begin.html [Accessed 25 January 2021].
8 Reuters. 'EU to Tighten Curbs Travel for Virus Hot Spots as Third Wave Fears Mount'. 21 January 2021. Available online at: www.reuters.com/article/us-health-coronavirus-eu-idUSKBN29Q1J1 [Accessed 25 January 2021].
9 euobserver. 'Portugal and Spain Under Pressure With Huge Covid Spike'. 29 January 2021. Available online at: https://euobserver.com/coronavirus/150759 [Accessed 1 February 2021].
10 DW. 'Coronavirus: Will EU Countries Close Borders Again?' 21 January 2021. Available online at: www.dw.com/en/coronavirus-will-eu-countries-close-borders-again/a-56298808 [Accessed 25 January 2021].
11 BBC News. 'Covid: How Are European Countries Tackling the Pandemic?'. 3 February 2021. Available online at: www.bbc.com/news/explainers-53640249 [Accessed 4 February 2021].

Bibliography

Alemanno, A., 2020. The European Response to COVID-19: From Regulatory Emulation to Regulatory Coordination? *European Journal of Risk Regulation*, 11(2), pp. 307–16.

Anderson, M., Mckee, M., and Mossialos, E., 2020. Covid-19 Exposes Weaknesses in European Response to Outbreaks. *BMJ* [e-journal] 368. https://doi.org/10.1136/bmj.m1075.

Aubrecht, P. et al., 2020. Centralized and Decentralized Responses to COVID-19 in federal systems: US and EU comparisons. *Law and Economics of Covid-19 Working Paper,* No. 4/2020 [online] Available at: http://dx.doi.org/10.2139/ssrn.3584182 [Accessed 20 January 2021].

Balmford, B. et al., 2020. Cross-Country Comparisons of Covid-19: Policy, Politics, and the Price of Life. *Environmental and Resource Economics*, 76, pp. 525–51.

Bargain, O. and Aminjonov, U., 2020. Trust and Compliance to Public Health Policies in Times of COVID-19. *Journal of Public Economics* [e-journal] 192. https://doi.org/10.1016/j.jpubeco.2020.104316.

Bénassy-Quéré, A. et al., 2020. Europe Needs a Catastrophe Relief Plan. In: R. Baldwin and B. Weder di Mauro, eds. *Mitigating the COVID-19 Economic Crisis: Act Fast and Do Whatever it Takes*. London: CEPR Press, pp. 121–8.

Bonardi, J.-P. et al., 2020. Fast and Local: How Did Lockdown Policies Affect the Spread and Severity of COVID-19? *CEPR Covid Economics Working Paper,* No. 23, [online] Available at: https://cepr.org/sites/default/files/news/CovidEconomics23.pdf [Accessed 19 January 2021].

Bouckaert, G. et al., 2020. European Coronationalism? A Hot Spot Governing a Pandemic Crisis. *Public Administration Review*, 80(5), pp. 763–73.

Brooks, E., de Ruijter, A., and Greer, S., 2021. Covid-19 and European Union Health Policy: From Crisis to Collective Action. In: B. Vanhercke, S. Spasova and B. Fronteddu, eds. *Social Policy in the European Union: State of Play 2020. Facing the pandemic*. Brussels: European Trade Union Institute. pp. 33–52.

Celi, C., Guarascio, D. and Somonazzi, A., 2020. A Fragile and Divided European Union Meets Covid-19: Further Disintegration or 'Hamiltonian Moment'? *Journal of Industrial and Business Economics*, 47, pp. 411–424. https://doi.org/10.1007/s40812-020-00165-8.

Coccia, M., 2020. Comparative Analysis of the First and Second Wave of the COVID-19: Is the On-going Impact of the Second Wave on Public Health Stronger than First One? *CocciaLab Working Paper,* No. 57/2020.

Deutsch, J., 2021. The EU's Coronavirus Vaccine Blame Game. Why So Slow? *Politico*, 4 January 2021. Available at: www.politico.eu/article/the-vaccination-blame-game-is-it-all-the-eus-fault/ [Accessed 25 February 2021].

Emiliani, T., 2020. How Relevant? The EU's 'Geopolitical' Commission and the Response to the Covid-19 Pandemic. *College of Europe Policy Brief*, No. 4.20 [online] Available at: http://aei.pitt.edu/102706/1/emiliani_cepob_4%2D2020.pdf [Accessed 20 January 2021].

European Commission, 2020. *EU Strategy for COVID-19 vaccines*. COM(2020) 245 final, 17 July 2020. Available at: https://eur-lex.europa.eu/legal-content/EN/TXT/PDF/?uri=CELEX:52020DC0245&from=EN [Accessed 8 February 2021].

Favero, C. A., Ichino, A. and Rustichini, A., 2020. Restarting the Economy While Saving Lives Under Covid-19. *CEPR Discussion Paper,* No. DP14664, [online] Available at: https://ssrn.com/abstract=3594296 [Accessed 20 January 2021].

Fetzer, T. R. et al., 2020. Global Behaviors and Perceptions at the Onset of the COVID-19 Pandemic. *NBER Working Paper,* No. 27082 [online] Available at: www.nber.org/papers/w27082 [Accessed 18 January 2021].

Gatto, M. et al., 2020. Speed and Dynamics of the Coivd-19 Epidemic in Italy: Effects of Emergency Containment Measures. *Proceedings of the National Academy of Sciences of the United States of America*, [e-journal] 117(19), pp. 10484–91. https://doi.org/10.1073/pnas.2004978117.

Goniewicz, K. et al., 2020. Current Response and Management Decisions of the European Union to the Covid-19 Outbreak: A Review. *Sustainability* [e-journal] 12(9), 3838. https://doi.org/10.3390/su12093838.

Graham, B. S., 2020. Rapid COVID-19 Vaccine Development. *Science* [e-journal] 368(6949), pp. 945–6. https://doi.org/10.1126/science.abb8923.

Grech, V., 2020. Unknown Unknowns – COVI-19 and Potential Global Mortality. *Early Human Development* [e-journal] 144. https://doi.org/10.1016/j.earlhumdev.2020.105026.

Greer, S. L., Ruijter, A. and Brooks, E., 2020. The COVID-19 Pandemic: Failing Forward in Public Health. In: M. Riddervold, J. Trondal and A. Newsome, eds. *The Palgrave Handbook of EU Crises*. London: Palgrave Macmillan, pp. 747–64.

Hervey, T., and Vanhercke, B., 2010. Health Care and the EU: The Law and Policy Patchwork. In: E. Mossialos et al., ed. *Health Systems Governance in Europe: The Role of EU Law and Policy*. Cambridge: Cambridge University Press, pp. 84–133.

Iserson, K. V., 2021. SARS-CoV2- (Covid-19) Vaccine Development and Production: An Ethical Way Forward. *Cambridge Quarterly of Healthcare Ethics*, 30, pp. 59–68.

Karnon, J., 2020. A Simple Decision Analysis of a Mandatory Lockdown Response to the COVID-19 Pandemic. *Applied Health Economics and Health Policy*, 18, pp. 329–31.

Kim, Y. C., B., Dema and Reyes-Sandoval, A., 2020. COVID-19 Vaccines: Breaking Record Times to First-in-Human Trials. *npj Vaccines* [e-journal] 5, p. 34. https://doi.org/10.1038/s41541-020-0188-3.

Middleton, J. et al., 2020. Planning for a Second Wave Pandemic of Covid-19 and Planning for Winter: A Statement from the Association of Schools of Public Health in the European Region. *International Journal of Public Health*, 85, pp. 1525–7.

Moreira, A. and Hick, R., 2021. COVID-19, the Great Recession and Social Policy: Is This Time Different? *Social Policy & Administration* [e-journal]. https://doi.org/10.1111/spol.12679.

Müller Gómez, J., and Thieme, A., 2020. The Appointment of the President of the European Commission 2019: A Toothless European Parliament? In: M. Kaeding, M. Müller, J., and Schmälter, eds. *Die Europawahl 2019*. Wiesbaden: Springer VS, pp. 181–90. https://doi.org/10.1007/978-3-658-29277-5_15.

Nicola, M. et al, 2020. The Socio-Economic Implications of the Coronavirus Pandemic (COVID-19): A Review. *International Journal of Surgery*, 78, pp. 185–93.

Oswick, C., Grant, D. and Oswick, R., 2020. Categories, Crossroads, Control, Connectedness, Continuity, and Change: A Metaphorical Exploration of COVID-19. *Journal of Applied Behavioral Science*, 56(3), pp. 284–8.

Pacces, A. M. and Weimer, M., 2020. From Diversity to Coordination: A European Approach to COVID-19. *European Journal of Risk Regulation*, 11(2), pp. 283–96.

Prudêncio, M., and Costa, J. C., 2020. Research Funding after Covid-19. *Nature Microbiology* [e-journal] 5, p. 986. https://doi.org/10.1038/s41564-020-0768-z.

Roberto, K. J., Johnson, A. F., and Rauhaus, B. M., 2020. Stigmatization and Prejudice during the COVID-19 Pandemic. *Administrative Theory & Praxis*, 42(3), pp. 364–78.

Schimmelfennig, F., 2017. Theorising Crisis in European Integration. In: D. Dinan, N. Nugent and W. E. Paterson, eds. *The European Union in Crisis*. London: Palgrave. pp. 316–35.

Schmidt, V. A., 2020. Theorizing Institutional Change and Governance in European Responses to the Covid-19 Pandemic. *Journal of European Integration*, 42(8), pp. 1177–93.

Sheikh, A. et al., 2020. What's the Way Out? Potential Exit Strategies from the COVID-19 Lockdown. *Journal of Global Health* [e-journal] 10(1), p. 010370. https://doi.org/10.7189/jogh.10.010370.

Stahl, A. K., 2020. Geopolitics in the Time of Coronavirus: The EU's Leadership in Global Health. *Hertie School – Jacques Delors Centre, Policy Position*, 9 June 2020, [online]. Available at: https://opus4.kobv.de/opus4-hsog/frontdoor/deliver/index/docId/3581/file/202000707_US_China_Relations_Stahl.pdf [Accessed 25 January 2021].

Uddin, S. et al., 2020. Onslaught of COVID-19: How Did Governments React and at What Point of the Crisis? *Population Health Management*, [e-journal]. http://doi.org/10.1089/pop.2020.0138.

Van Schaik, L., Jørgensen, K. E. and van de Pas, R., 2020. Loyal at Once? The EU's Global Health Awakening in the Covid-19 Pandemic. *Journal of European Integration*, 42(8), pp. 1145–60.

Verhofstadt, G., 2021. I Love the EU – But the Vaccine Strategy Is a Fiasco. *euobserver*, 16 February 2021. Available at: https://euobserver.com/stakeholders/150931 [Accessed 16 February 2021].

Vesan, P., Corti, F., and Sabato, S., 2021. The European Commission's Entrepreneurship and the Social Dimension of the European Semester: From the European Pillar of Social Rights to the Covid-19 Pandemic. *Comparative European Politics* [e-journal] 19(6). https://doi.org/10.1057/s41295-020-00227-0.

Veugelers, R. and Zachmann, G., 2020. Racing against COVID-19: A Vaccines Strategy for Europe. *Bruegel Policy Contribution,* No. 07/2020 [online] Available at: www.bruegel.org/wp-content/uploads/2020/04/PC-07-2020-210420V3.pdf [Accessed 21 January 2021].

Von der Leyen, U., 2020d. Press Statement by European Commission President, Ursula von der Leyen on the market authorization of the BioNTech/Pfizer vaccine against COVID-19. 21 December 2020. Available at: https://audiovisual.ec.europa.eu/en/topnews/M-006027 [Accessed 8 February 2021].

Von der Leyen, U., 2021. Speech by President von der Leyen at the European Parliament Plenary on the state of play of the EU's COVID-19 vaccination strategy, 10 February 2021. Available at: https://ec.europa.eu/commission/presscorner/detail/en/speech_21_505 [Accessed 16 February 2021].

Wolff, S. and Ladi, S., 2020. European Union Responses to the Covid-19 Pandemic: Adaptability in Times of Permanent Emergency. *Journal of European Integration*, 42(8), pp. 1025–40.

6 Constitutionalising the state of exception

Implications for citizenship

6.1 Introduction

Constraints to the mobility of citizens were decided at the national level, when national governments realised the contagious potential of the virus and hence forced citizens into lockdown. National governments resorted to the state of exception, causing the temporary disavowal of some fundamental rights. Constitutional exceptionalism was grounded on the urgency to alleviate the spread of the virus. It is a breach of constitutional guarantees afforded to citizens, but this is hardly envisaged as a breach of the Constitution (at least by authors who legitimised the state of emergency).

A deeper review is necessary, though. There was no consensus on constitutional exceptionalism as the strategy to contain the virus by forcing citizens' reclusion. Critics claim that proportionality was not respected, and the state of exception was premature and not reasoned. The unintended effects of the state of exception with constitutional backup are at stake for the future. Critics acknowledge that formal mechanisms act as a protection against the abuses of constitutional exceptionalism. Parliaments have the final say on the approval of the state of exception. The institution that directly represents citizens decides whether citizens must endure restrictions on fundamental rights for the sake of a superior goal. Maybe this is not enough, especially when governments increasingly take a recourse to exceptions to temporarily undermine fundamental values.

The issue bears importance for European integration. One fundamental value of European integration is the rule of law and fundamental rights assigned to citizens by the constitutional settlement. It must be remembered that the EU turned into a legal provision of its own the respect of the rule of law and fundamental individual rights when examining whether applicant countries are eligible to the EU membership (Ethier, 2003). As in the previous two chapters, however, decisions approved at the national level have an impact on European integration. Needless to say, EU institutions have no responsibility, nor do they have a say, when a country ponders the possibility of enforcing constitutional exceptionalism. Still, the EU is not disconnected from member states and, indeed, member states still play an influential role in

DOI: 10.4324/9781003153900-7

the configuration of EU policies. Thus, the question is whether constitutional exceptionalism also hampers the EU.

The research hypothesis is whether the contamination of the EU by constitutional exceptionalism must be disregarded because of the broader sense of exceptionalism triggered by the pandemic. Non-conventional approaches of law are added to the analysis. They move within a different analytical framework. The awareness that non-conventional sources of law come to the forefront, and that they are linked to the volatile nature of law in response to changing social circumstances, brings a new scenario to the analysis. This innovative analytical framework must be compared with the conventional model of constitutionalism and to the strict obeyance to the rule of law, and whether, for both approaches, constitutional exceptionalism is acceptable as a precondition for the adjustment of the legal system to temporary anomalies that strike the society. The EU cannot escape this discussion, not only for the embeddedness on the rule of law, but also because the EU has a legal system with many formal and substantial similarities with member states' legal systems (Martinico and Pollicino, 2012). The threat comes from the perception that the EU might be forced to accept constitutional exceptionalism at a certain moment for reasons outside its political willingness, since the state of exception is an outcome of national governments' decisions only.

The chapter proceeds as follows. Section 1 elaborates on the justifications provided by governments when they enforced the state of exception. Section 6.2 turns to the critics of constitutional exceptionalism. Of particular relevance is the reasoning they put forward about the disproportionality between the means and ends. Section 6.3 addresses the opposite stance: to what extent the state of exception was inescapable, considering the emergency raised by the pandemic and the need to mitigate the transmission of the virus? For this purpose, the consensus on constitutional exceptionalism is anchored on legal pluralism that encompasses a flexible hermeneutic of constitutional provisions. Section 6.4 asks whether the spirit of European integration, notably the adherence to the foundations of the rule of law and the prevalence of constitutionally embedded rights, was challenged by constitutional exceptionalism, and to what extent it is detrimental for the EU.

6.2 The rationale of the state of exception

When national governments realised that lockdown was the precondition to mitigate the propagation of COVID-19, legal measures were devised to provide a robust legal background to lockdown. Considering that restraints to persons' circulation needed strong legal support, countries resorted to the utmost exceptional measure at their disposal: the state of exception that allows to temporarily derogate individual freedoms on grounds of exceptional circumstances that cannot be immediately addressed otherwise (Zinn, 2020).

The trade-off between civil liberties and constraints upon them is generally encompassed on national Constitutions under the heading of the state of exception (Dyzenhaus, 2006). With some variations from country to country (minor variations, though, as the basic precept of the rule of law cuts across all member states and the EU itself), special provisions are included in Constitutions laying down the formal requirements to enact the state of exception and what is the maximum impact on citizens' freedoms. National governments were asked to substantiate the state of exception on a twofold criterion (Greene, 2020):

i from the *formal point of view*, procedures written on constitutional provisions concerning the implementation of the state of exception were strictly followed;
ii from the *substantial point of view*, they decided the restrictions to be introduced to the freedom of circulation so that citizens would be confined to their houses for a certain period of time.

The rationale of the state of exception was beyond doubt for national authorities. The correlation between the colossal contagious potential of COVID-19 with public health concerns (not to mention a vast array of second order implications, starting with the economy) brought the state of exception to the table. A negative trade-off was found between preserving basic civil liberties (notably the freedom of circulation within the country, not to mention across countries) and fighting the dissemination of the virus. Alarmed with the quick spread of the disease and the difficult situation in which hospitals were in, governments were pushed to the limit. Challenged with exceptional circumstances that eroded the routine societies were used to, governments had to take a difficult decision. The only possibility was to impose restrictions on people's mobility as a way to restrain the proliferation of the virus and relieving hospitals from the pressure they were put under (Plümper and Neumayer, 2020).

At the outset of the pandemic, member states were battered by the virus in different ways. This explains why different degrees of constitutional exceptionalism were implemented (Balmford et al., 2020). An extended state of exception was decided where COVID-19 took more lives and affected more persons in relative terms (Italy, Spain, France), while others implemented soft versions. Countries severely hit by the first wave of the pandemic resorted to comprehensive lockdown, forcing the population in general to an extensive curfew. Only selected categories of persons were allowed to come into the streets, whenever they were working in economic sectors deemed necessary to people's subsistence as well as in hospitals, police forces and state institutions with a critical input on the crisis management. Correspondingly, severe restrictions with a legal background were designed to force persons to stay at home. Episodes of police strict monitoring and legal action taken against citizens not respecting the state of exception were documented (Conteduca et al., 2020; Terpstra et al., 2021). In countries less affected by COVID-19 a milder version of the state of exception was introduced (Yan et al., 2020). Curfew was not so tight and individual circulation was tolerated to a certain extent. The state of exception was not so harsh, and corresponding legal measures to enforce the state of exception were less stiff.

The early experience with legal provisions that implemented the state of exception afforded skills to national governments when countries were struck by the second and the third waves of the pandemic. The capital of experience was important not only on the public health dimension of the pandemic crisis (how to address the new challenges of the virus, notably when different strains were added to the pandemic) but also to the political dimension attached to the decision of how and when to enforce the state of exception, as well as to the appropriate legal measures. The public health and the political and legal dimensions cannot be untied. The state of exception was envisaged as the last resort solution to tame the contagious effects of the pandemic crisis (Bouckaert et al., 2020). Constitutional exceptionalism was instrumental to the sanitary dimension of the crisis.

The recognition of how constitutional exceptionalism was instrumental to the pandemic crisis management brings another issue to the discussion. The political decision that endorsed the state of exception should be solidly grounded on constitutional terms, both for the procedural requirements and for the justification. Thus, communication was a sensitive issue. Governments realised that the fulfilment of legal procedures supporting the state of exception might not be enough, as the plea to constitutional exceptionalism also required a robust, coherent legitimacy background (Schraff, 2020). Cutting off citizens' basic rights was a critical decision. Hence, in addition to the formal requirements following constitutional provisions on the state of exception, governments should pay attention to the justification of measures that curtailed citizens' rights by forcing them to curfews of variable degrees (Baldwin, 2021).

The articulation between political communication and legitimacy is of paramount importance when authorities resort to constitutional exceptionalism and enforce restrictions to basic civil liberties. Citizens will be willing to comply with the state of exception as long as they are given persuasive arguments on the necessity of exceptional measures. Forcing persons to stay home, imposing strict limits to go outside and submitting citizens to police monitoring when they walk in the streets is a contradiction to the principles that govern modern liberal democracies. The outcome of political action is exceptional, as the underlying conditions that justify constitutional exceptionalism. The scope for a thorough, well-grounded justification of the state of exception is more demanding that the need to secure citizens' consent supporting ordinary political decisions (Reeskens and Muis, 2020).

There is mixed evidence of the articulation between political communication and legitimacy when national governments resorted to the state of exception more than once (Former and Kohler, 2020). The challenges authorities faced were overwhelming. They were compelled to action by the urgency of addressing the thorny effects of the sanitary crisis, but they also had to deal with the sensitive issue of enforcing and justifying the state of exception. The connection with the input and the output dimensions was paramount. Constitutional exceptionalism of this kind was a challenge to the democratic regime, the rule of law and citizens' basic rights (Belling, 2020). Although the conditions that paved the way to the state of exception were exceptional in themselves, the decision and its communication were decisive for governments' strategy as far as an effective crisis management was concerned.

6.3 Criticisms of constitutional exceptionalism

The implementation of the state of exception was widespread. No member state of the EU escaped what governments judged to be an inevitable decision. The potential of contagion of COVID-19 was exponential and, hence, the pandemic was escalating. The sense of disarray predominated. National authorities, based on scientific expertise, realised that exceptional measures were necessary in order to mitigate the contamination and the rise of the death toll. This is the underlying narrative of the political decision that forced lockdown and the corresponding constraints on fundamental rights regarding free mobility.

The reaction to the state of constitutional exceptionalism was not undivided. Amidst forbearance, as if the majority of citizens was convinced by national authorities' rhetoric, some voices rallied against lockdown and the underlying rationale. Above all, critics were not certain on whether lockdown was the right reaction to fight the dissemination of COVD-19 (Boretti, 2020). They claimed that the sudden decision to restrict people's freedom of circulation was not mature. For that purpose, governments' swift action was pointed out as the shortcoming of the widespread resort to lockdown (Robinson, 2021). More scientific evidence was needed, despite the acceleration of the pandemic with the implications observed (the rising number of people infected and increasing casualties, as well as the turmoil that was hitting national healthcare systems).

For critics, the re-hierarchisation of means and ends became salient. For the mainstream approach to the sanitary crisis, means were instrumental to the urgency of the ends. Critics also realised that the sense of urgency triggered governments to a political rationale consistent with the exceptionality societies were faced with. Although critics recognised this was the official narrative, they disputed it (Warren et al., 2021). The articulation between means and ends in the political arena, especially when means are sacrificed in order to fulfil the ends, thus elevating the latter to the utmost priority, must be carefully assessed. Such assessment was largely absent, according to critics. The decision to address the challenges of the mounting pandemic was prone to the chaos that contaminated societies and to the need to quickly drain the dissemination of the contagious virus. At this point, governments did not hesitate in sacrificing the means (free mobility of persons) and protecting the ends (to reverse the pandemic). For national governments, the anaesthesia of citizens' free mobility was instrumental to the main goal of halting, as much as possible, the development of the pandemic. The consequence of anaesthetising citizens' mobility was their hibernation (Tisdell, 2020).

Critics, however, did not voice against the procedural aspects of the state of exception approved in member states (and elsewhere). Procedural requirements to enforce the state of exception were respected everywhere (Guruparan, 2020). The involvement of national parliaments granted a veil of democratic legitimacy to the process. In spite of constitutional proceduralism not being jeopardised, the criticism was directed at the substance. They were not convinced by the underlying rationale of constitutional exceptionalism. More important than recognising that the input towards the state of exception was respected is the discussion of substantial aspects that justify the option for constitutional exceptionalism. The critics' position was that no compelling reasons justified the state of exception. Two positions came forward against the narrative of the unavoidable lockdown based on constitutional exceptionalism.

The first argument points out the untenable concession of civil liberties to the economy (Žižek, 2020). After some inaction, when governments were faced with the first signs of the pandemic, they quickly reacted, one after the other, with the implementation of radical measures that limited the freedom of mobility and threatened to spread poverty. Apparently, governments' underlying narrative emphasised the prevalence of sanitary concerns over economic concerns. They argued citizens should stay at home to avoid the dissemination of the virus. Apparently, as well, political authorities dodged in favour of the preservation of public health and were not concerned about the functioning of the economy. People should stay home even if that involved sacrificing the economy. The economy could wait until the sanitary crisis did not bite as hard. The image that ostensibly emerges is governments more worried with people's health condition than with the economy. A scale of priorities was unravelled to the outsider, the a-critical consumer of governmental communication: public health comes before the economy when a dreadful pandemic threatens to spread death and pain.

The official rhetoric must nevertheless be submitted to thorough examination. Appearances can be deceptive. The starting point of the analysis is the systemic intentionality that permeates the functioning of the capitalist system (Žižek, 2020). The genetic imprint of the capitalist template influences political authorities. They are prone to the interests of large companies that dominate production at the worldwide level and not so much to the interests of the large majority of consumers and workers (Peters, 2020). There are plenty of manifestations of this biased approach on the Western world. For this reason, the question about intentionality makes sense. Behind the veil of political communication, is anything different hidden? This where the meeting with systemic features of the capitalist system takes place. Although political communication pointed out to the prevalence of public health concerns over the functioning of the economy, exceptions were granted to what governments considered priority sectors of activity. In addition, an unusual (for current standards) organisation of the labour market was enacted, giving rise to homeworking and lay-off mechanisms. The economy was not sacrificed as it seemed (Ali, 2021).

Keeping persons at home was not a measure dictated by public health considerations only. The immediate goal was to mitigate the dissemination of the virus, hence creating conditions for preventing more damage to public health and the public healthcare system. At the same time, systemic features of the capitalist system cannot be ignored to the point of asking whether governments were thinking in the economy as the non-immediate goal. Despite failing to be recognised by mainstream analysis, the economy was also being preserved by forcing persons to stay at home (Toscano, 2020). A devastating pandemic would claim many more lives. A higher death toll would involve long-term implications to the functioning of the economy. Restricted markets (both because of the considerable number de casualties and of income cuts) lead to decreasing consumption, forcing companies to decrease production and to cut their massive profits. In addition, higher the number of deaths the more the production capacity of companies could be affected.

This is a cynical analysis: political authorities were eager to preserve human lives as much as possible to the extent that such option was crucial to the medium- to long-term preservation of the economy (Žižek, 2020). Yet, according to the critics, governments themselves concealed their rhetoric with cynicism. At the outset of the pandemic, when disarray was the nightmare for political authorities and the learning effects of the fight against the virus were not accessible, governments' narrative was about the protection of human lives and public health. If they threw the economy into the table, it was only to discuss what kind of exceptional economic policy ought to be designed to cushion the negative implications of the pandemic on the economy.

Intentionality (tied to the systemic features of the capitalist system) is the background of the criticism against constitutional exceptionalism. The deeper reasons underlying the state of exception are not grounded on genuine concerns with the preservation of human lives. Governments' bias in favour of capitalism, especially of large and influential companies, provides the rationale of constitutional exceptionalism (Di Cesare, 2020). Governments were ready to sacrifice basic individual rights not because they were concerned with saving lives, but because that was instrumental to the medium- to long-term protection of the economic system (Dias and Deluchey, 2020).

The second line of reasoning against constitutional exceptionalism on the pandemic days is anchored to the semi-perennial state of exception argument (Agamben, 2021). The Italian philosopher stood out as one prominent theoriser of the state of exception (Agamben, 2005). The earlier Agamben was already concerned with the mutability of constitutional rules when the state of exception is enforced. He warned that the incorporation of constitutional provisions stipulating the preconditions to endorse the state of exception was no guarantee that the exception became the rule, and the rule was turned into an exception. Even in democratic states, where strong guarantees to the strict enforceability of the rule of law exist, the danger of disruption existed. He also realised that special circumstances require special measures, which, in turn, might be consistent with constitutional exceptionalism, as long as political justification is convincing among political actors and the majority of citizens, and formal requirements allowing the declaration of the state of exception are obeyed.

Agamben returned to the theorisation of the state of exception when governments all over the world decided to impose severe constraints on the mobility of people and, for that purpose, announced the state of exception. His analysis was controversial, as some authors diverged not only from Agamben's criticisms to the state of exception but also from his reasoning (e.g., Swiffen, 2012). This time, Agamben was suspicious that the implementation of the state of exception was not a genuine necessity, even though the challenges of the sanitary crisis were sizeable. He condemned 'the growing tendency to use the state of exception as a normal governing paradigm'

Again, it was time to dispute the hierarchy between means and ends, with a different reasoning. The severity of the sanitary crisis and the need to mitigate the spread of the virus by forcing lockdown was not an acceptable argument to lay down constitutional exceptionalism. Agamben envisaged the race to lockdown like a race to the bottom on the rule of law and the compliance with basic individual rights.

The state of exception was more a manifestation of authority, especially important in times of exceptional circumstances that require harsh measures that curtail basic personal rights. This tendency follows the constant pattern of 'crisification' (in Europe and elsewhere) as the precondition to enforce exceptions to the legal system of democratic states insomuch as the stability of the system is prone to exceptions that gradually interrupt rules. More and more, exceptions become the rule and the rule is the exception (Salter, 2005). In Agamben's interpretation, the gradual evolution of democratic regimes to easily encompass constitutional exceptionalism entails a corruption of the rule of law and of democracy. In times where democratic legitimacy increasingly shifted from the input to the output dimension, the rise of the state of exception, and how straightforwardly democratic governments resort to it, confirms this modern layer of corruption to the way democratic legitimacy is assessed. Means must be sacrificed when political authorities estimate that an outcome is the priority that faces no obstacles. Procedures are twisted when needed by taking stock of hermeneutic flexibility or by arguing that in the face of emergency only exceptional measures are available. This tendency is consistent with the misrepresentation of democracy, bringing democratic regimes closer to the constitutional anomaly that is typical of non-democratic regimes or the so-called 'illiberal democracies' (Kádár, 2020).

The threat comes from the re-signification of democracy through what Weiler (2020) dubbed the 'self-asphyxiation of democracy'. When democracy tolerates the widespread corruption of constitutional provisions that protect basic individual rights, or when democracy is congruent with the corruption of the rule of law when in a growing number of cases exceptions become the rule, democracy (at least from the point of view of mainstream, liberal democracies understanding) is at stake. The swift state of exception that unfolded in Europe and many other countries in the first wave of the pandemic seems to have maximised this tendency so that it is difficult to understand where the genuine nature of democracy lies.

Subsequent events, notably the political reaction of national authorities to the second and the third waves of the pandemic by forcing citizens to lockdown again, seem to confirm Agamben's pessimistic analysis. Constitutional exceptionalism during the first wave of the pandemic opened the window of opportunity for the ensuing future state of exception motivated by the considerable worsening of the pandemic (Scheppele and Pozen, 2020). Together with the learning effects of the evolution of the pandemic, all that was necessary was to fine tune the state of exception to the changing conditions of the pandemic and to communicate convincingly. Structural inertia paved the way for new waves of the state of exception based on how the first wave of constitutional exceptionalism was enacted and on the overall consensus among stakeholders and citizens about the imperative of lockdown when the number of contaminated persons and casualties rose impressively.

This criticism shares, to a certain extent, the rationale of systemic intentionality. Agamben's scepticism on the modern evolution of democracies is the theoretical background (Murphy, 2021). Ongoing constitutional exceptionalism is understood as a corruption of democracy, of how democratic leaders and practitioners surrender to the silent temptation of authoritarianism (Dezalay, 2020). This source of authoritarianism differs from the one proclaimed by right-wing populist parties, though. The continuing route to constitutional exceptionalism adds an element of uncertainty that is not congruent with long-established guarantees of the rule of law. Citizens are increasingly aware that they must submit to exceptions to the constitutional settlement whenever the country is under the radar of turmoil. Increasingly as well, citizens get used to the manifestations of authority of political authorities that easily evaporate into the distortion of democracy (Lührmann and Rooney, 2020). What is difficult to prove (not to mention, impossible) is to what extent the recurrent use of the state of exception is an outcome of political actors' intentionality.

The two arguments against the normalisation of constitutional exceptionalism are internally similar on what concerns the recognition of embedded systemic intentionality. They diverge on the sources that trigger the corruption of democracy through the normalisation of the state of exception. While Žižek sees the permeability of democracy to the influences exerted by capitalism, Agamben shifts the focus to political actors' behaviour, putting the blame for the corruption of democracy on them. They have in common the perception that constitutional exceptionalism was ill-designed and lacks robust arguments. For that reason, the critics conclude that constitutional exceptionalism lacked democratic legitimacy and acts as a source of erosion of democratic regimes (Arato, Claussen and Heath, 2020).

6.4 A legal pluralist rationale of constitutional exceptionalism

Legal pluralism thrives in the analysis of legal and political issues (Davies, 2010). It is particularly important when the issues at stake have a legal connection, so that the analytical tools required apparently come from law. Yet, law does not exist in isolation. Legal systems are shaped by political decisions that judge multifaceted aspects that organise the society (history, sociology, psychology, legal structures, political foundations, the international context that influences the legal system as well). Thus, a flexible, transdisciplinary approach is considered the first-best solution (Melissaris, 2016). The analysis and the hermeneutic exercise transcend law, as the legal system is permeable to inputs coming from other social sciences. The methodological approach is plural to the extent that encompasses other social sciences in addition to law. The epistemological turn to legal pluralism acknowledges that law is not hostile to the evolution of social conditions as well (Berman, 2009). Open-ended analysis is necessary in order to capture the nature of social phenomena that might ask for changes in legal provisions.

Legal pluralism accepts the reconfiguration of legal provisions when special circumstances change the context for their implementation (Melissaris and Croce, 2017). For that purpose, flexible interpretation is a possibility. In times when changing basic rules of the legal system is not an option, but where different challenges arise from special conditions outside law, the solution comes from the adjustment of legal provisions. The legal system is permeable to open-ended provisions that, in turn, easily accommodate to new circumstances whenever such flexibility is not detrimental to the nature of the political system itself and basic political and constitutional values are not threatened.

The possibility of constitutional exceptionalism is not envisaged as a threat to democracy and the rule of law. On the one hand, the legal system encapsulates formal requirements that must be followed when special conditions call for a flexible interpretation or for temporary derogation of constitutional provisions. Hence, as long as procedural requirements are met and special conditions legitimise exceptionality, no corruption of the rule of law, and of the legal system, takes place (Kysela, 2020). On the other hand, the interpretation of events that might call for temporary suspension of constitutional provisions (or at least for their flexible interpretation) relies on the consensus that emerges among political actors and citizens. In other words, the focus shifts to how convincing political communication is when the justification of constitutional exceptionalism is at stake (Bishai, 2020). The issue of legitimacy is quintessential for accepting temporary derogations to constitutional provisions.

This is where supporters of legal pluralism and critics of constitutional exceptionalism diverge. Legal pluralism is comfortable with the possibility of constitutional flexibility in the face of exceptional circumstances, as long as the basic canons of the political and legal system are not under stress and political communication is convincing. Differently, critics do not accept that persuasive political communication is a substitute of formal rules, as this solution could entail a threat to democracy. If formal guarantees enshrined in the constitutional settlement are softened and give way to political communication, the legal system is superseded by political communication. Rhetoric, as convincing as it might be, is not a substitute of legal rules. Rhetoric encompasses a huge degree of subjectivism, thereby denying one feature of the legal system: stability that comes from an objective understanding and implementation of legal rules. Law, and legal, positive hermeneutics provide an element of continuity and stability, adding to the stability of the political system (Tuori, 2016), which the vagaries of political communication is not able to deliver.

For legal pluralism, the key to understand why constitutional exceptionalism was necessary during the pandemic lies on the re-hierarchisation of ends and the accommodation of means. The narrative is somewhat different from the one suggested by the critics of the state of exception. The latter emphasise that ripped basic rights based on the declaration of the state of exception is an anomaly of means and ends, as ends become the priority and they supersede means, carving their hibernation. Legal pluralism is not totally opposed to the critics' rationale. Their supporters agree that ends must comply with means. Nonetheless, means must accommodate to the ends in exceptional cases that require exceptional measures (Menski, 2014).

This approach points out how pragmatism pushes political actors to sway in favour of ends and to adjust the means accordingly. Pragmatism pegs to the rationale of weighting alternative outcomes in the face of expected consequences tied to the alternatives. When alternative interpretations of available means come into the equation, a pragmatic approach picks the costless when the relevant variables are estimated. For a comprehensive analysis of the challenges of the pandemic, the alternatives were:

i to strictly abide by the founding principles that grant citizens' fundamental rights and recognise that the underlying context of the quick dissemination of the disease was not powerful enough to put the ends ahead of the means. Therefore, conditions to enforce the state of exception were not met; or

ii to consider that the urgency of the pandemic was the evidence of how circumstances turned into exceptional, opening the window of opportunity to give the goal (the mitigation of the pandemic) superiority over the means (citizens' fundamental rights). Constitutional exceptionalism was grounded on how exceptional were the conditions that affected the world. Corresponding adjustment of means (temporary exceptions to the freedom of movement) did not entail a sacrifice of democracies' basic values neither a re-parameterisation of the rule of law.

For legal pluralism, the incorporation of the manifold variables to the political analysis of the sanitary crisis pushed for pragmatism. The uncertainty of the pandemic closed the doors to experimentalism, as it could involve an unbearable price in terms of casualties, turmoil on public health, healthcare system disarray, with additional side effects on many other areas (economic crisis, political instability, social unrest, and so forth). Supporters of legal pluralism were not ready to pay that high price because human lives are priceless (Delanty, 2020). In order to protect the superior value of human life, they were ready to temporarily sacrifice basic human rights in the name of the successful mitigation of the pandemic. Furthermore, as long as the decision to enact the state of exception complied with procedural requirements, at least the rule of law was not jeopardised.

For these reasons, legal pluralism was prone to the second scenario mentioned above. The combination of facts and the awareness of why individual rights should undergo temporary neutralisation to foster a successful reversal of COVID-19 shed light on the methodology of legal pluralism. Instead of giving rise to substantive aspects, as the opponents of constitutional exceptionalism did (what lies underneath the decision to curtail basic individual rights?), legal pluralism paid attention to a pragmatic, formalistic approach. Their supporters were not concerned with finding undisputable justifications in favour of the state of exception. They relied on the prevailing uncertainty and took a pragmatic stance that helped to envisage constitutional exceptionalism as the inevitable leap forward in the comprehensive strategy to defeat the pandemic. Since they were convinced of the overwhelming potential of the pandemic, and of how lockdown was necessary to curb the progression of the virus, their reasoning was consistent with exceptional, temporary restrictions to people's freedom of movement. Constitutional exceptionalism would entail no damage to the rule of law and to the genetic imprint of liberal democracies.

The divergence between supporters of legal pluralism and opponents of constitutional exceptionalism lies on the diagnosis of the hierarchy between means and ends. For the critics, the acritical acceptance of the state of exception involves a re-hierarchisation of ends and means, as the latter are sacrificed to meet the former. Legal pluralists disagree with the diagnosis. They argued that a temporary derogation of some civil liberties (notably the freedom of movement) is imperative to meet the higher goal – to tame the pandemic (Nyamutata, 2020). This process is a deep wound on basic values of liberal democracies. Instead of viewing the outcome as a re-hierarchisation of ends and means, legal pluralism suggests a different combination: in order to meet the ends, a temporary adjustment of means is pictured. The uniqueness of events that spread disarray and threatened to kill more people legitimised the rearrangement of priorities and the ensuing temporary scaling down of means.

What remains to be seen is whether hidden scars get tattooed in the skin of societies. Critics of constitutional exceptionalism fear that the window of exceptionality was easily broken, thereby breaching conventional preconditions to an exceptional regime as far as civil rights is concerned. This is an important source of opposition coming from critics to constitutional exceptionalism: the precedent is too serious to be neglected. They fear that constitutional exceptionalism becomes embedded, not only among policymakers but also (and especially) among apathic citizens, so that in the future it will be easier to resort to the state of exception with minor scrutiny from the citizenry (Kuo, 2020; Bishai, 2020).

6.5 Where does the European Union stand amidst constitutional exceptionalism?

The declaration of the state of exception lies among national governments' exclusive competences (White, 2021). Hence, whether the EU is affected by the imperative of constitutional exceptionalism that at some point emerged when countries and the EU were dealing with the pandemic seems to be meaningless. EU institutions have no say on why, when and how to enforce the state of exception.

Yet, the analysis is not so simple as the confirmation of the assignment of competences might reveal. European integration brings the supranational and national levels increasingly embedded. Despite some layers of policy-making kept reserved to the exclusive competences of national governments, this does not entail the absence of the EU on some of these issues, sometimes acting as an external observer that, nevertheless, 'names and shames'. What is important to account is that the EU is a polity with embedded constitutional values and constitutional provisions that matter for the issue at stake. Not only the EU promotes freedoms of movement, one of the genetic footprints of European integration, but the Union was given its own charter of fundamental rights (Coman, 2020). Notwithstanding the national level is autonomous to decide the state of exception, the possibility that national decisions that temporarily curtail basic individual rights clash against EU's fundamental values and constitutional provisions makes the EU an interested actor on national decisions.

What matters here is not the unfinished controversy about the priority of legal orders, whether the EU law as a whole is superior to member states' legal orders or not (outside those areas of uncontested recognition of the primacy of EU law, such as regulations and directives over national laws). For the purposes of this section, the relevant discussion is not about the problematic relationship between national Constitutions and EU's constitutional provisions, notably when they offer conflicting solutions. When looking to the competence to enforce the state of exception, the delimitation of powers between the EU and member states rules out any dispute.

Yet, national governments' implementation of the state of exception encompassing provisions that contradict basic constitutional values of the EU add another layer of complexity. It is important to emphasise what is at stake: it is not a conflict between two sources of constitutional provisions, it is a conflict between the choice of constitutional exceptionalism by the national level and the non-compliance of basic values of the EU as a consequence of the national decision. There is no formal conflict between both legal systems. The conflict that deserves inspection is the lack of congruence between constitutional exceptionalism at the national level and the ontology of European integration. Two questions come to the surface: considering that the EU and member states are enmeshed, does the state of exception enforced at the national level obstruct basic constitutional values of the EU? Does this paradoxical status hinder the EU as a polity that guarantees basic freedoms that, in turn, were temporarily suspended at the national level?

The testable hypothesis is whether the absence of overseeing powers of the EU on member states' compliance with constitutional values, notably those that guarantee fundamental rights, is a weakness that becomes salient in exceptional times. In normal times, member states and the EU act as protectors of fundamental rights (Fabbrini, 2014). The EU obeys to a genetic imprint that emphasises democracy and human rights as core values. Member states are the first shield against the disruption of such values. National constitutional settlements and long-term political stability with the prevalence of mainstream centre-right and centre-left parties in governments both worked in favour of the rootedness of these values (Streeck, 2017). The maintenance of this coalition becomes problematic when emergency hits the ground, for the absence of means for EU institutions to closely monitor whether temporary derogations of fundamental values are consistent with member states' constitutional procedures.

Although special procedures for judging member states when they act against democracy and the rule of law are enshrined in the EU constitutional settlement (Article 7, Treaty on the European Union), past experience shows how punishment is unlikely. First, unanimous voting is required to approve a decision regarding punishing a member state that walks away from democratic values or the rule of law. Second, recent experience is straightforward about negative coalitions of member states preventing unanimous voting from taking place. That is the case of the attempts to bring Hungary accountable for breaching the values stated in Article 2 of the Treaty on the European Union and how other Visegrád countries blocked the attempt.[1] Importantly, the initiative took place before the pandemic, during 'normal times', when a strict compliance of the rule of law and the respect for democratic values was likely to be consensual among national governments.

European integration faces a conundrum. The EU is a reference for democracy, the rule of law and the protection of fundamental human rights (Schimmelfennig, 2010).[2] Indeed, the EU is stringent on these values when a country submits the application to the EU (Conant, 2014). Also, these are the political conditions for the EU to deliver development aid to developing countries (Koch, 2015). Despite all its flaws, the EU constitutional settlement includes the possibility of imposing sanctions on member states that threaten democracy or fail to comply with the rule of law or do not fully respect human rights. In theory, the EU is a champion of democracy, the rule of law and the protection of human rights (Meunier and Vachudova, 2018). What is problematic is the internal consistency of such theoretical underpinnings with practice when normal times are replaced by exceptional constitutionalism. Without an overseeing role on member states' resort to the state of exception, the EU is prone to weaknesses. Guarantees that democracy and the rule of law are not overshadowed, or that temporary exemptions to basic human rights fail to meet the criterion of proportionality and justification, are especially important when exceptionality assumes centre stage. It is in hard times that fundamental values face increasing risks of non-compliance, not in routine years.

The conundrum must be set into the context of European integration. The autonomy of the EU is recognised. However, member states still play a pivotal role in the course of action, be it through political oversight exerted by the European Council or by regular decision-making in the Council. In addition, the EU is meaningless if it could be thought in isolation of member states (Bickerton, 2012). The conundrum is only a theoretical exercise considering the current distribution of powers between the EU and national authorities. Nevertheless, the exercise is not hollowed out. A discussion on the implications of the paradoxical consequences of constitutional exceptionalism for European integration must not be avoided. Otherwise, the passive acceptance of 'things as they are' puts the EU against the wall.

The EU has no means to circumvent the possibility that member states walk away from democracy, the rule of law and the protection of fundamental human rights other than the flimsy provision written on Article 7 of the Treaty on the European Union. Outperformed by member states' doubtful resort to the state of exception, the EU is not able to reinstate values compromised by the excesses of national governments. This affects the democratic performance of the EU, one way or another. Needless to say, the EU is not to blame for member states' deviations. Yet, since member states are endogenous to the functioning of the EU, when they hurt democracy, the rule of law or basic civil rights, they make the EU their collateral victim.

On the other hand, we recognise that a changing pattern would involve a revolutionary outcome for which national authorities are not prepared for (at the time of writing). Granting EU institutions an overseeing role on national governments' compliance of these values would entail a radical departure from how European integration is currently shaped. It would definitely mean more Europe – maybe too much Europe for the political willingness of today's national governments, bearing in mind the sensitive political cycle in which we live in. This additional weakness of the EU heightens the conundrum. The gap between desirability and feasibility is noticeable. At the end of the day, the EU is 'innocently guilty' when shortcuts to democracy, the rule of law and the protection of human rights are observed at the national level (Lacey and Nicolaïdis, 2020).

Important questions emerge from the previous analysis: was the EU temporarily stripped away of one founding value (the freedom of mobility across member states) when national governments resorted to constitutional exceptionalism on grounds of the strategy to overcome the pandemic? In urgent cases that require exceptional measures (such the enforcement of the state of exception that temporarily derogates the freedom of mobility), is the EU surpassed by member states, thereby showing a weakness of the EU?

The first question puts in the antagonism between critics of constitutional exceptionalism and the supporters of legal pluralism. The answer depends on the stance the reader takes. It is easy to grasp arguments that invalidate or corroborate the resort to the state of exception and, hence, provide a negative assessment for European integration or to conclude that the EU's stamp of free mobility was not jeopardised (respectively). The awareness that persons' mobility was severely restricted, not only across member states but also within each member state, is perhaps the evidence that European integration suffered no harm. The problem was not temporarily stripping away the EU from a fundamental value, but to understand the underlying reasons and to also recognise that restrictions to mobility were first and foremost domestic and, by implication, EU-wide as well (Lebret, 2020).

The second question is more sensitive. Gradualism is the keyword to understand the history of European integration. Although the EU enjoys a considerable degree of autonomy, it is still far away from total autonomy as member states still play a pivotal role. In addition, the organisation of the political system where the EU and member states overlap shows how political oversight and the key to ordinary legislation still remain at the mercy of the national level (Müller, 2015). Faced with an urgent situation that required urgent crisis management, together with the seriousness of the contagious potential of COVID-19, national governments realised that lockdown was the solution to at least stop the dissemination of the virus. Ultimately, putting obstacles to people's mobility at the national level does not threaten freedom of movement as a fundamental value of the EU (see Chapter 4). At the same time, to consider that the EU was offset by the national level is misleading. The EU has no jurisdiction on member states' territorial units when their governments acknowledge the urgency of confining citizens at home.

6.6 Conclusions

According to national governments and to those who supported the state of exception, constitutional exceptionalism was a crucial step forward in the strategy to mitigate the pandemic. Notwithstanding exceptional circumstances were the underlying reason to temporarily suspend individual rights such as the freedom of movement, important questions arise as to how convincing the reasoning about the inevitability of the state of exception was (Hantrais and Letablier, 2021). At the same time, thorough scrutiny of procedural requirements was a precondition to legitimise constitutional exceptionalism. Not everybody was convinced of the need to enforce the state of exception. Actually, many challenged the underlying intentions and the legitimacy of the state of exception.

The rift between supporters and critics of constitutional exceptionalism is something positive that came through the pandemic crisis. Amidst mayhem and people's panic, there was space for discussion. Despite some political actors asking for a united front against the pandemic, thereby suggesting that political confrontation characteristic of democracy should be temporarily deferred, there was room for a battle of ideas and an exchange of arguments. At least the virus was not able to amputate ideas, as the contestation to constitutional exceptionalism and its theoretical background showed. It was, at the same time, an important proof of life of how citizens were not under the pandemic's anaesthesia that could have thrived some sort of civic hibernation. If that were the outcome, another layer of disease (cutting off non-mainstream arguments) would add to the main layer – the effects of COVID-19.

This raises another important implication of constitutional exceptionalism: the consequences for citizenship. On the one hand, obvious implications emerged from the state of exception, as citizens' fundamental rights underwent temporary suspension. If, however, the underlying arguments of constitutional exceptionalism are accepted, as well as the observation of formal requirements and the mantle of legitimacy fed by proper communication to citizens, the damage to citizenship rights was the inevitable price to pay for the strategy to overcome the pandemic. On the other hand, at a deeper level, even if the necessity of the state of exception is accepted and how the adjustment of means to the end was unavoidable, the temporary suspension of fundamental civil rights must be duly noted. For what matters, a sanitary crisis was so powerful that in order to mitigate the propagation of the virus the freedom of movement was temporarily interrupted, forcing societies to go back to the medieval age when simply crossing from one town to another was forbidden.

The pandemic was an attack on citizenship, as well. At the same time, it raised fundamental challenges to political actors, at the national and the EU level. Faced with the chaos resulting from the pandemic, the output of the political process was more important than ever. A proper adjustment to the sanitary crisis (and to the other crisis that followed) required expertise and diligence about the strategy to mitigate COVID-19. To that extent, the pandemic raised a twofold challenge to citizenship: citizens relied on the quality of political outcomes to smooth suffering and the number of casualties as well as the accommodation to the challenges of the pandemic; but they also should closely monitor the outcomes of the political process, not only to judge the efficiency of political decisions but also to consider exceptional circumstances that might soften a critical judgement of political actors.

Notes

1 Reuters. 'Eastern EU States Tell Brussels to Back Off'. 26 January 2018. Available online at: www.reuters.com/article/us-europe-hungary-visegrad-idUSKBN1FF1U3 [Accessed 12 March 2021].
2 For a contrasting perception (on how the EU damaged democracy), see Scharpf (2015).

Bibliography

Agamben, G., 2005. *State of Exception*. Chicago, IL: University of Chicago Press.

Agamben, G., 2021. *Where Are We Now? The Epidemics as Politics*. London: Eris Press.

Ali, S., 2021. Žižek, Agamben and the Idea of Democratic Biopolitics. *Review of Human Rights*, 6(1), pp. LXV–LXXIII. https://doi.org/10.35994/rhr.v6i1.157.

Arato, J., Claussen, K. and Heath, J. B., 2020. The Perils of Pandemic Exceptionalism. *American Journal of International Law*, 114(4), pp. 627–36.

Baldwin, P., 2021. *Fighting the First Wave: Why the Coronavirus Was Tackled So Differently Across the Globe*. Cambridge: Cambridge University Press.

Balmford, B. et al., 2020. Cross-Country Comparisons of Covid-19: Policy, Politics, and the Price of Life. *Environmental and Resource Economics*, 76, pp. 525–51.

Belling, V., 2020. The State of Exception and Limits of the Rule of Law. In: J. Jinek and L. Kollert, ed. *Emergency Powers: Rule of Law and the State of Exception*. Baden-Baden: Nomos, pp. 43–74.

Berman, P. S., 2009. The New Legal Pluralism. *Annual Review of Law and Social Science*, 5, pp. 225–42.

Bickerton, C. J., 2012. *European Integration: From Nation States to Member States*. Oxford: Oxford University Press.

Bishai, L. S., 2020. The Inertia of Exception. In: L. S. Bishai, ed. *Law, Security and the State of Perpetual Emergency*. London: Palgrave Macmillan, pp. 11–36.

Boretti, A., 2020. After Less Than 2 months, the Simulations That Drove the World to Strict Lockdown Appear to be Wrong, the Same of the Policies They Generated. *Health Services Research and Managerial Epidemiology*. https://doi.org/10.1177/2333392820932324.

Bouckaert, G. et al., 2020. European Coronationalism? A Hot Spot Governing a Pandemic Crisis. *Public Administration Review*, 80(5), pp. 763–73.

Coman, R., 2020. Democracy and the Rule of Law: How Can the EU Uphold its Common Values? In: R. Coman, A. Crespy and V. Schmidt, ed. *Governance and Politics in the Post-Crisis European Union*. Cambridge: Cambridge University Press, pp. 358–77.

Conant, L., 2014. Compelling Criteria? Human Rights in the European Union. *Journal of European Public Policy*, 21(5), pp. 713–29.

Conteduca, F. et al., 2020. Fighting Covid-19: Measuring the Restrictiveness of Government Policies. *Banca d'Italia Covid-19 Note*, 27 May 2020, [online]. Available at: www.bancaditalia.it/pubblicazioni/note-covid-19/2020/Nota_Lockdown_circolazione.pdf [Accessed 8 March 2021].

Davies, M., 2010. Legal Pluralism. In: P. Cane and H. M. Kritzer, ed. *The Oxford Handbook of Empirical Legal Research*. [online]. Available at: https://doi.org/10.1093/oxfordhb/9780199542475.013.0034 [Accessed 10 March 2021].

Delanty, G., 2020. Six Political Philosophies in Search of a Virus: Critical Perspectives on the Coronavirus Pandemic. *LSE Europe in Question Discussion Paper Series*, No.156/2020, [online] Available at: www.lse.ac.uk/european-institute/Assets/Documents/LEQS-Discussion-Papers/LEQSPaper156.pdf [Accessed 8 March 2021].

Dezalay, S., 2020. Introduction: Wars on Law, Wars through Law? Law and Lawyers in Times of Crisis. *Journal of Law and Society*, 47(S1), pp. S1–13.

Di Cesare, D., 2020. *Virus Sovrano? L'Asfissia Capitalistica*. Torino: Bollati Boringhieri.

Dias, B. L. C. V. and Deluchey, J.-F. Y., 2020. The "Total Continuous War" and the COVID-19 Pandemic: Neoliberal Governmentality, Disposable Bodies and Protected Lives. *Law, Culture and the Humanities*. https://doi.org/10.1177/1743872120973157.

Dyzenhaus, D., 2006. *The Constitution of Law: Legality in a Time of Emergency*. Cambridge: Cambridge University Press.

Ethier, D., 2003. Is Democracy Promotion Effective? Comparing Conditionality and Incentives. *Democratization*, 10(1), pp. 99–120.

Fabbrini, F., 2014. *Fundamental Rights in Europe. Challenges and Transformations in Comparative Perspective*. Oxford: Oxford University Press.

Former, L. and Kohler, J. C., 2020. Global Health and Human Rights in the Time of COVID-19: Response, Restrictions, and Legitimacy. *Journal of Human Rights*, 19(5), pp. 547–56.

Greene, A., 2020. *Emergency Powers in a Time of Pandemic*. Bristol: Bristol University Press.

Guruparan, K., 2020. Constitution and Law as Instruments for Normalising Abnormalcy: States of Exception in the Plurinational Context. In: R. Albert and Y. Roznai, ed. *Constitutionalism Under Extreme Conditions: Law, Emergency, Exception*. Heidelberg: Springer, pp. 63–79.

Hantrais, L. and Letablier, M.-T., 2021. *Comparing and Contrasting the Impact of the Covid-19 Pandemic in the European Union*. London: Routledge.

Kádár, A., 2020. In Its Nature – How Stealth Authoritarianism Keeps Stealing Along During the Pandemic, and How Can it be Stopped? *Journal of Human Rights Practice*, 12(2), pp. 293–300.

Koch, S., 2015. A Typology of Political Conditionality Beyond Aid: Conceptual Horizons Based on Lessons from the European Union. *World Development*, 75, pp. 97–108.

Kuo, M.-S., 2020. From Institutional Sovereignty to Constitutional Mindset: Rethinking the Domestication of the State of Exception in the Age of Normalization. In: R. Albert and Y. Roznai, ed. *Constitutionalism Under Extreme Conditions: Law, Emergency, Exception*. Heidelberg: Springer, pp. 21–39.

Kysela, J., 2020. Exceptionality in Law. In: J. Jinek and L. Kollert, ed. *Emergency Powers: Rule of Law and the State of Exception*. Baden-Baden: Nomos, pp. 101–24.

Lacey, J. and Nicolaïdis, K., 2020. Democracy and Disintegration: Does the State of Democracy in the EU Put the Integrity of the Union at Risk? In: R. Coman, A. Crespy and V. Schmidt, ed. *Governance and Politics in the Post-Crisis European Union*. Cambridge: Cambridge University Press, pp. 378–97.

Lebret, A., 2020. COVID-19 Pandemic and Derogation to Human Rights. *Journal of Law and the Biosciences*, 7(1). https://doi.org/10.1093/jlb/lsaa015.

Lührmann, A., and Rooney, B., 2020. Autocratization by Decree: States of Emergency and Democratic Decline. *Comparative Politics*, [e-journal]. https://doi.org/10.5129/001041521X16004520146485.

Martinico, G. and Pollicino, O., 2012. *The Interaction between Europe's Legal Systems: Judicial Dialogue and the Creation of Supranational Laws*. Cheltenham: Edward Elgar.

Melissaris, E., 2016. *Ubiquitous Law: Legal Theory and the Space for Legal Pluralism*. London: Routledge.

Melissaris, E. and Croce, M., 2017. *A Pluralism of Legal Pluralisms*. Oxford Handbooks Online. Available at: https://doi.org/10.1093/oxfordhb/9780199935352.013.22 [Accessed 10 March 2021].

Menski, W., 2014. Remembering and Applying Legal Pluralism: Law as Kite Flying. In: S. P. Donlan and L. H. Urscheler, ed. *Concepts of Law: Comparative, Jurisprudential, and Social Science Perspectives*. Farnham: Ashgate, pp. 91–108.

Meunier, S. and Vachudova, M. A., 2018. Liberal Intergovernmentalism, Illiberalism and the Potential Superpower of the European Union. *Journal of Common Market Studies*, 56(7), pp. 1631–47.

Müller, J.-W., 2015. Should the EU Protect Democracy and the Rule of Law inside Member States? *European Law Journal*, 21(2), pp. 141–60.

Murphy, M. P. A., 2021. The Double Articulation of Sovereign Bordering: Spaces of Exception, Sovereign Vulnerability, and Agamben's Schmitt/Foucault Synthesis. *Journal of Borderland Studies*, 36(4), pp. 599–615. https://doi.org/10.1080/08865655.2019.1683053.

Nyamutata, C., 2020. Do Civil Liberties Really Matter During Pandemics? Approaches to Coronavirus Disease (COVID-19). *International Human Rights Law Review*, 9(1), pp. 62–98.

Peters, M. A., 2020. Philosophy and Pandemic in the Postdigital Era: Foucault, Agamben, Žižek. *Postdigital Science and Education*, 2, pp. 556–61.

Plümper, T., and Neumayer, E., 2020. Lockdown policies and the dynamics of the first wave of the Sars-CoV-2 pandemic in Europe. *Journal of European Public Policy*. https://doi.org.10.1080/13501763.2020.1847170.

Reeskens, T. and Muis, Q., 2020. A New Democratic Norm(al)? Political Legitimacy amidst the Covid-19 Pandemic. In: Aarts, E., et al., ed. *The New Common: How COVID-19 Pandemic is Transforming Society*. Tilburg: Tilburg University Press, pp. 189–94.

Robinson, O., 2021. COVID-19 Lockdown Policies: An Interdisciplinary Review. *SSRN*, 9 February 2021 [online] Available at: http://dx.doi.org/10.2139/ssrn.3782395 [Accessed 9 March 2021].

Salter, M. B., 2005. At the Threshold of Security: A Theory of International Borders. In: E. Zureik and M. B. Salter, ed. *Global Surveillance and Policing: Borders, Security, Identity*. Portland: Willan, pp. 36–50.

Scharpf, F. W., 2015. After the Crash: A Perspective on Multilevel European Democracy. *European Law Journal*, 21(3), pp. 384–405.

Scheppele, K. L., and Pozen, D., 2020. Executive Overreach and Underreach in the Pandemic. In: M. P. Maduro and P. W. Kahn, ed. *Democracy in Times of Pandemic: Different Futures Imagined*. Cambridge: Cambridge University Press, pp. 38–53.

Schimmelfennig, F., 2010. The Normative Origins of Democracy in the European Union: Toward a Transformationalist Theory of Democratization. *European Political Science Review*, 2(2), pp. 211–33.

Schraff, D., 2020. Political Trust during the Covid-19 Pandemic: Rally around the Flag or Lockdown Effects? *European Journal of Political Research*. https://doi.org/10.1111/1475-6765.12425.

Streeck, W., 2017. The Rise of the European Consolidation State. In: H. Magara, ed. *Policy Change under New Democratic Capitalism*. London: Routledge. pp. 27–46.

Swiffen, A., 2012. Derrida Contra Agamben: Sovereignty, Biopower, History. *Societies*, 2(4), pp. 345–56.

Terpstra, J. et al., 2021. Policing the Corona Crisis: A Comparison between France and the Netherlands. *International Journal of Police Science & Management*, 23(2), pp. 168–81. https://doi.org/10.1177/1461355720980772.

Tisdell, C. A., 2020. Economic, Social and Political Issues Raised by the Covid-19 Pandemic. *Economic Analysis and Policy*, 68, pp. 17–28.

Toscano, A., 2020. The State of the Pandemic. *Historical Materialism*, 28(4), pp. 3–23.

Tuori, K., 2016. *Critical Legal Positivism*. London: Routledge.

Warren, G. W. et al., 2021. COVID-19: The Winter Lockdown Strategy in Five European Nations. *Journal of Risk Research*, 24(3–4), pp. 267–93. https://doi.org/10.1080/13669877.2021.1891802.

Weiler, J. H. H., 2020. COVID, Europe, and the Self-Asphyxiation of Democracy. In: M. P. Maduro and P. W. Kahn, ed. *Democracy in Times of Pandemic: Different Futures Imagined*. Cambridge: Cambridge University Press, pp. 141–52.

White, J., 2021. Emergency Europe after Covid-19. In: Delanty, G., ed. *Pandemics, Politics and Society: Critical Perspectives on the Covid-19 Crisis*. Berlim: Walter de Gruyter, pp. 75–92.

Yan, B. et al., 2020. Why Do Countries Respond Differently to COVID-19? A Comparative Study of Swede, China, France, and Japan. *The American Review of Public Administration*, 50(6–7), pp. 762–9.

Zinn, J. O., 2020. 'A Monstruous Threat': How a State of Exception Turns into a 'New Normal'. *Journal of Risk Research*, 23(7–8), pp. 1083–91.

Žižek, S., 2020. *Pandemic! COVID-19 Shakes the World*. New York: OR Books.

Conclusion

The EU as a crisis manager in the pandemic – good but not great

In March 2020, the world woke up to a pandemic crisis that had been silently forming in the last months of 2019. What had began to be dismissed by the European and international technical authorities as a 'low-risk' problem rapidly escalated to a major global crisis, with multiple layers (sanitary, economic, political, social) that severely impacted citizens' daily life and led governments worldwide to adopt unprecedented measures to halt the spreading of the virus. In this book we attempted a first assessment of the role of the EU as a crisis manager in the first year of the pandemic. It is, thus, a provisional assessment, considering how volatile the development of the pandemic and the adjustment of political authorities (in the EU and elsewhere) have been. When we planned to write a book on the EU's management of the COVID-19 pandemic we couldn't imagine that one year later the ensuing multidimensional crisis was far from being solved. After all, the input of uncertainty, the DNA of COVID-19 evolution, was the biggest obstacle we had to overcome during the writing process.

Our central argument is that, despite similarities with previous crises (such as the Eurozone or the migration crises), COVID-19 has a fundamental difference, as it is a symmetric crisis. This symmetry, we claim, should boost cooperation between the EU member states. If our argument is to be proven, we expected to see a preference for a response to the crisis devised at the supranational level (a European *common* response) over individual, unilateral decisions and actions (*national* responses).

We were also interested in seeing if and how the pandemic opened a window of opportunity for changing EU policies and procedures. The bourgeoning literature on crisis acknowledges that crisis could represent a critical juncture that enables a moment of transformation in long periods of stability. However, the crisis-reform thesis is also challenged by reality. The literature shows that more often than expected, after an early claim for reform, political leaders are keener to return to the status quo than to advance deep institutional or policy reforms. Considering that the COVID-19 pandemic exposed the fragilities of several policy areas, both at the national and the EU level, we have attempted to highlight and assess the changes that have occurred (or were proposed) as a result of the crisis. For this purpose, we resorted to an adaptation of

DOI: 10.4324/9781003153900-8

the Streeck and Thelen model (2005). The authors draw attention to the fact that change could result either from abrupt processes (such as crisis) therefore resulting in breakdown and replacement (discontinuity), or from incremental processes, leading to incremental change (continuity). Our proposal is that a crisis could also lead to boosted incremental change (a push forward). The literature that studied crises in the EU is conducive to this reasoning. Also, considering that EU's policies and decision-making process involve several actors, frequently with fundamental differences as regards their agendas and preferences, a significant difference between the proposal (the type of change envisioned) and the decision approved (the type of change that actually occurs) takes place.

Building on the above-mentioned framework (explored in Chapter 1), we have started by broadly examining the politics of the pandemic (Chapter 2). We looked at the interplay between the national and the international levels in the response to the multiple layers of the crisis. By tracing the process from January 2020 to early April 2021, we managed to identify patterns of cooperation and non-cooperation. We then zoomed in on the economic dimension of the crisis (Chapter 3), highlighting the effects in the EU's economy and assessing the solutions proposed at the EU level. In the following chapters, the book addressed the sectoral analysis of the crisis by assessing the consequences of the restrictions to free movement (Chapter 4), by evaluating the sanitary and humanitarian dimension (Chapter 5), and by problematising the state of exception (Chapter 6). Our aim was to answer one central research question (devised in the Introduction): *Did the EU perform well as a crisis manager in the initial stages of the pandemic crisis?* Since this is a broad, evaluative question, we defined five subsidiary research questions that also guided the research:

(i) Was economic policy consistent with the challenges stemming from the crisis?
(ii) Did the pandemic trigger an institutional recalibration of the EU institutional system?
(iii) Was it possible to overcome national unilateralism and bring the EU to the centre stage?
(iv) Did exceptionalism (border controls, humanitarian emergency feeding national reassurance, and constitutional exceptionalism) hinder European integration? If so, are negative implications bound to be transitory?
(v) In the current state of the pandemic, do we have more Europe or less Europe?

At this point, a note of caution is due. Our analysis took place during the first year of an ongoing crisis. Therefore, our conclusions are necessarily preliminary, as the frequent use of the expression 'at the time of writing' throughout the book indicates. Also, measuring change goes well beyond the analysis of the proposals, even if the process of adoption is already concluded. Indeed, a look at the phases of implementation and evaluation is key to assess the type and degree of change. Notwithstanding, bearing in mind the timeframe of this investigation this is not a possibility. Therefore, the robustness of our conclusions has to be checked against the test of time.

On the politics of the pandemic, our findings suggest that at the early stages of the crisis the EU was unable to secure a visible central role, therefore failing to shape the initial response to the COVID-19 crisis. Several factors might help to explain this understated performance: when the first case of COVID-19 was reported from a European country there was very limited information regarding the pace of spreading and the severity of the virus that was first reported in Central China; previous health threats raised an alarm among international and European authorities, but ended up having much more moderate effects in Europe than initially anticipated, which might account for some optimistic biases regarding COVID-19 disease; indeed, at the outset the international authorities, namely WHO, had toned down the severity of the threat, and so did the EU technical bodies that were monitoring the problem; the EU has very limited competences in health policy and although there are crisis management structures in place, the mandate and interoperability of those structures was not robust enough; in January 2020, the new Commission had roughly one month in office (Ursula von der Leyen replaced Jean-Claude Juncker on 1 December 2019), so the normal reorganisation of the Commission's services was most likely in course; on the issue of the appointment of the new Commission, some authors point out, in addition, that the abandonment of the *spitzenkandidaten* process might have affected the political visibility of the institution when it came into office.

Regardless of the reasons, and despite the close monitoring of the problem by the technical bodies, the EU missed the opportunity to be prepared when the crisis hit Europe, therefore failing one crucial crisis management task: preparedness. The EU also missed the opportunity to take the lead as regards sense-making, that is, understanding and explaining the COVID-19 crisis. Despite having a specialised agency in disease control (the ECDC), the EU left the early framing of crisis narrative in the hands of member states. The result was an initial period of profound disarray, in which member states' governments reacted using an 'every man for himself' strategy. This inward-looking stance prevented national leaders from paying attention to the symmetry of the crisis, and therefore, unilateral action and competitiveness were preferred over concerted action and cooperation. In the eyes of the critics, the EU's apparent slip worked as a self-fulling prophecy: a disunited Europe responded to the crisis in disunion. Considering that the support for a political system has always a utilitarian dimension,[1] this raised questions regarding the purpose (and the durability) of the European integration project.

As the crisis unfolded, and the effectiveness of uncoordinated action became manifest, the EU's role steadily increased. The narrative changed accordingly.

Coordination became the most repeated word in EU institutions' crisis-related documents as well as in the speeches of EU leaders (at the supranational but also at the national level). Gradually, a shift from unilateral action to the use of institutionalised cooperation took place through a coordinated response to the crisis. The Commission embodied the coordinator role, first by using the SM banner, but afterwards by responding to the direct call of other EU institutions. By creating or seizing existing opportunities, the Commission framed the crisis narrative, constructed an image of efficiency and union and played a central role in crisis management. However, reputation is a fragile asset, as the hurdles of EU's vaccine campaign showed. The ECB, under a new leadership, confirmed the proactive stance that adopted during the last stage of the Eurozone crisis, expressing a position that resembled Draghi's 'do whatever it takes' attitude. The European Council, although taking a back seat, met frequently to closely monitor the EU's response.

When the issues on the negotiation table were perceived as having big payoffs, as it was the case of the negotiations of the MFF or the related recovery and resilience plan, some member states did not hesitate to put cooperation aside to engage in strict intergovernmental bargaining, which resembled 'business as usual' despite the urgency of the response to the ongoing crisis. That being said, many decisions were adopted at an unusual rapid pace, which seems to confirm the idea advanced by Rhinard (2019), who pointed to a 'crisification' of the decision-making process. This pattern might account for the apparent low profile of the EP in crisis response, which is also explained by the lockdowns that limited the regular functioning of the European assembly, particularly during the first wave of the pandemic. The EP did however make abundant use of other tools, such as hearings.

On the question of institutional recalibration, our findings suggest that the pandemic crisis did not significantly alter the EU institutional balance. The Commission continued a trend (noticeable during the Juncker Commission) of reasserting its political role, thus casting serious doubts on previous accounts on the institution's irrelevance. Actually, in the contest between winners and losers the Commission would have been the clear winner, was not for the controversy surrounding the negotiations with AstraZeneca. The European Council, though with less visibility, maintained tight control of the process of crisis response. The ECB confirmed the relevance of its action, particularly to ease the reactions of the financial markets and to provide a buffer to the economic policy accommodation of the crisis. The EP was, at first sight, a victim of the 'crisification' process, although the parliament managed to explore competences other than its legislative role in order to get involved in the crisis response process. Assuming that dealing with successive crises is the 'new normal', the EP needs to explore alternative forms of participation (other than its crucial, but less visible in crisis situations, legislative role), if it wants to appear in the winners' team. As co-legislator, the role of the Council was also limited by the urgency of the response. As normally happens in situations of crisis, the work of the Council is outshined by the mediatic attention given to European Council meetings, the natural forum for political leadership.

When we break down the analysis and focus on the specific dimensions of the crisis, the findings confirm this global assessment. As the sanitary dimension of the crisis escalated and lockdowns were imposed to try to halt the spread of the virus, the economic layer of the crisis emerged. The shutdown of non-essential economic activities severely affected production and consumption. Data collected regarding the first half of 2020 shows an abrupt fall of GDP and a decline of employment rates, even though the overall impact of the crisis on the market job was mitigated by exceptional measures implemented early on. That being said, the number of jobs that were lost is far from being negligible. What is more, the most fragile groups of the labour market (youngsters, women, temporary workers) were the most affected ones.

The increase of social inequality confirms a pattern usually seen in crisis situations, substantiating the need to pay particular attention to the groups that are already prone to exclusion in normal times. The economic downturn also impacted on member states' public finances, echoing memories of the previous sovereign debt crisis. Unlike what happened then, this time the EU was quick to intervene. After some weeks of unilateral responses, member states finally switched to a coordinated response at the European level, although some individual states occasionally gained prominence. Several proposals to mitigate the economic effects of the crisis were negotiated, including an ambitious recovery plan. The adoption of the proposals occurred at an impressive pace confirming that, after some hesitation and despite (concerning) manifestations of national egoism, cooperation through policy coordination was the preferred path to deal with the economic dimension of the crisis.

The exceptional circumstances opened the door for a paradigm shift not only as regards economic policymaking, but also regarding economics per se. As already happened in previous crisis (although for a short period of time), a Keynesian-inspired economic policy emerged as the appropriate solution to prevent the devastating effects of the economic collapse in the short run and to stimulate economic recovery in the medium term. However, whether this represents a permanent teleological shift away from the monetarist, ordoliberal template of economic policymaking that influenced EMU or simply a temporary, pragmatic move that policymakers endorsed for as long as the exceptional circumstances last is yet to be seen. Perhaps reports of a paradigm shift on economic policymaking, as well as categorical judgements of how market failures became palpable and how the government is indispensable, are partial and premature. Time, again, will tell whether the scar tissue of the pandemic crisis resonates in the medium to long term and whether the skin of societies will be different as a consequence of the woes of COVID-19. At this moment, no one can tell if normality (as we knew it before the pandemic crisis) will be back again. It is understandable that moderation and caution should guide the hermeneutics of the pandemic crisis.

Understandably, one persistent aspect in the COVID-19 pandemic crisis response was the use of exceptionalism. Border closures is another example. Despite the lack of scientific evidence (at the beginning of the crisis neither the WHO nor the EU technical bodies recommended border closures), one of the first non-medical countermeasures that member states resorted to stop the pandemic was to reinstate internal border controls. As a consequence, European citizens' right to free movement was severely hampered. EU member states' reaction was not abnormal. Confronted with an unfamiliar security threat that menaced the survival of the state, governments reacted in a familiar way, by closing their borders. The early response of member states to the COVID-19 pandemic was therefore a classic example of the securitisation process. The health problem was perceived and framed as a security threat by securitisation agents (national leaders, the media, the scientific community), which in turn opened the door for the use of extraordinary protection measures (including border closures). The generalised use of war-type rhetoric was illustrative of this securitisation process. Once the issue was securitised, the adoption of severe restrictions to the mobility of European citizens, with the broad support of the citizens whose rights were restricted, was facilitated.

The securitisation of COVID-19 raised important questions, particularly regarding legitimacy and the long-term consequences of the limitations imposed on citizens' mobility. Freedom of movement has been a building block of the European integration process since the beginning. Although initially dependent on the economic activity of the person, it rapidly evolved to become a central principle of the European way of life. Whereas national citizenship has a fixed territorial component, European citizenship is built around the idea that European citizens are free to move across Europe. The Schengen agreement created a borderless area that enabled this idea. COVID-19 suspended mobility. Sure, it was not the first-time internal borders were closed. The terrorist attacks in some European countries or the migration crisis have both being used to trigger SBC exceptional clauses and their successive extensions.

However, the level of restrictions justified by the need to stop the spreading of the virus was unprecedented, thus fuelling the debate about the legitimacy of the measures adopted. If we approach the legitimacy problem through the acceptance of authority's lens, it seems fair to argue that the measures adopted by national governments were perceived as legitimate, since a significant part of the population accepted that mobility restrictions were needed to stop the transmission of the virus. However, legitimacy has a legal basis, meaning that the measures adopted should conform to the law. This entails passing the necessity, proportionality and non-discrimination tests, which was not exactly the case. Although the scientific evidence points to a reduction of the level of transmission, provided mobility restrictions were generalised, it was not clear that member states were able to comply with the 'burden of proof', that is, to provide evidence of the absolute necessity of the measures imposed. The scale, pace and strictness of the measures adopted across Europe also significantly varied, and they did not apply uniformly to all European citizens, which raised red flags regarding both proportionality and non-discrimination principles.

These doubts were echoed by the European institutions that repeatedly reminded the importance of free movement and steadily claimed for re-opening Europe as the control of pandemic appeared to be on track. A decrease in the numbers of the infected people allowed a process of de-securitisation. The idea of gradually returning to 'normality' dominated the EU's narrative. However, after a cooling off period in the number of infections, European states experienced second and third waves of the COVID-19 crisis and new restrictions to mobility were reinstated as a response. This time, however, the adoption of the measures was less haphazard. Some level of EU coordination was already in place. Also, since the de-securitisation process was in motion in the end of the first wave, the scrutiny of the measures adopted during the second and third waves increased and the importance to list clear and objective criteria, based on scientific evidence, to justify restrictions to citizens' rights became vital. Additionally, citizens' tacit agreement and compliance with the restrictions became less generalised, suggesting that early large acceptance of border restrictions was contingent to the severity of the pandemic. It was just the outcome of a sense of vulnerability and of the perception that limits on free movement were important to stop the dissemination of the virus, and not a sign of a fundamental shift in the way EU citizens value freedom of movement.

The severity of the crisis brought the necessity of humanitarian emergency. Since the crisis began as a sanitary crisis, to reinforce the resources allocated to public healthcare systems (hospitals staff and facilities, public health lines, medicines, equipment) was among national authorities' first priorities. Initially, the emphasis was on national reassurance. However, some early competitiveness showed that disarticulated responses would most likely result in competitions putting one member state against the other, which ultimately could jeopardise the overall purpose of the European project. The coordination at the EU level that followed prevented would-be fratricide rivalries.

A paradigmatic shift was the decision to engage on joint procurement to buy COVID-19 vaccines and to devise a Europe-wide vaccination campaign. We do realise that the EU vaccination strategy faced several hurdles. At the time of writing (early April 2021) the process is not yet at full steam and several setbacks have been noticed. As the EU trailed back to the UK or the United States, many blamed the inexperience of the Commission in this type of negotiations, EU's red tape and the cumbersome, time-consuming EU's decision-making process. Our findings suggest that the Commission is hardly the only one to blame for delays in the EU's vaccination campaign. Factors such as pharmaceutical companies' profit calculations, difficulties in the mass production of vaccines, problems in supply chains, concerns about some side effects of the vaccines have all to be considered. Also, the EU can only act within the limits of the competences that the 27 member states conferred upon it. In practice, this means that any development that fosters the role of the EU needs the consent of national governments. Interestingly, Chancellor Merkel recognised in late April 2021 that the EU needs to be given a prominent role as far as a genuinely effective EU health policy is concerned.[2] Thus, a direct comparison between the EU and a sovereign state is misleading.

The biggest example of exceptionalism was the extended use of the state of exception by member states. The idea was to guarantee a strong legal support to the adoption of crisis responses that severely restricted some citizens' rights. Paradoxically, however, for some the declaration of the state of exception suffered from legal and legitimacy problems, as it was neither sufficiently justified, nor proportional. Critics of constitutional exceptionalism argued that the state of exception was the perfect subterfuge to squeeze citizens' rights considering the challenges of the pandemic crisis. Yet, they were not convinced that the state of exception was justified, despite the fact that procedural requirements were met. According to the critics, constitutional exceptionalism was just a disguise of 'business as usual', with the difference that the pandemic gave political authorities a veil of legitimacy when they decided to restrict citizens' rights. The book addressed two strands of this critical approach: one based on the assumption that the systematic features of capitalism prevailed once again and, therefore, restrictions laid down by governments were consistent with saving the economy and large companies' preferences; another that examined the current state of constitutional exceptionalism as just the outcome of an ongoing trend that spreads the confusion between means and ends, between rules and exception, pointing out that the rule becomes the exception and the exception is transfigured into the rule.

The analysis of a contrasting approach brought indeterminacy into the discussion. Supporters of constitutional exceptionalism provided the rationale for the state of exception given the background of a persistent and uncertain pandemic crisis. They realised that the end at stake (to curb the dissemination of COVID-19) should be given absolute priority. Hence, a temporary derogation of available means (the existing constitutional system) was accepted, not only because the articulation of means and ends showed, this time, that the former should be temporarily sacrificed for the sake of the latter, but also because the constitutional requirements of the state of exception were met. Exceptional circumstances allowed for a soft reinterpretation of constitutional guarantees. For supporters of constitutional exceptionalism, the imminent tragedy of the pandemic provided the veil of legitimacy for the state of exception.

The constitutional analysis of the COVID-19 pandemic has a legal-philosophical dimension embedded, which, nevertheless does not exhaust the ramifications of the issue at stake. Questions concerning the seeming apathy of EU institutions, on the one hand, and to what extent might constitutional exceptionalism be considered a setback to the fundamental values of European integration, on the other hand, came to the surface. Notwithstanding the idea of a powerlessness EU emerged – and, what is worse, how the state of exception upsets EU's genetic imprint of freedom of movement – the conclusion deserves some qualifications, since the issue at stake lies within the exclusive powers of national authorities.

What are the implications of this sectoral analysis for the broader argument of the book? Our findings partially confirm our central argument concerning cooperation. At the early stage of the pandemic, each government ignored the symmetric nature of the crisis, treating the threat as a national problem (or even for some time as someone's else problem) that would require national solutions, instead of a common threat that should have a common response. However, it did not take too long until member states were confronted with the symmetry of the crisis. The rapid spreading of the virus across Europe (and worldwide) made it clear that no member state would escape the pandemic, even if the pace of the crisis varied. Member states thus accepted to replace uncoordinated, unilateral actions by a crisis response coordinated at the European level.

The awareness that uncooperative moves hinder effectiveness, leading to suboptimal results, seems to have played a part in this shift. EU institutions, particularly the Commission, carefully constructed a narrative emphasising the need for coordination and the perils of disarticulated responses. An effective communication strategy and a clear chain of command are well-known assets in situations of crisis and the Commission seized the opportunity to take on the coordination role. The Commission's narrative was also instrumental in countervailing disinformation regarding the EU crisis response that was feeding the 'global battle of narratives'[3] (Borrel, 2021) within and outside the EU. Certainly, COVID-19 crisis management revealed a number of fragilities in response capacity, not only at the national level but also at the EU level. But an overall assessment of the EU performance in crisis response strongly contradicts the image of a helpless Europe that was widely disseminated in the early stages of the pandemic. On the contrary, our findings suggest that by praising and enabling cooperation, the EU was able to play a central role in crisis management. The EU has also taken a leading role in promoting cooperative solutions for the crisis globally.

In what refers to change, the COVID-19 crisis offered (and keeps on offering) a unique laboratory for policy learning based on the assessment of mistakes and failures, but also of the best practices in crisis response. The cascading effects of COVID-19 crisis had an impact on several policy areas, creating the right momentum for policy change. According to the Commission's 2020 Strategic Foresight,[4]

> [i]n light of the COVID-19 crisis and of the transition-led political agenda, it is clear that Europe needs to further strengthen its resilience and bounce forward, i.e., not only recover but emerge stronger by intensifying these transitions. The EU needs to draw lessons from the pandemic,

anticipate future developments, and strike the right balance between the wellbeing of current and future generation.

(European Commission, 2020, p. 6)

Besides proposals to respond to immediate or foreseen effects of the pandemic, several proposals aimed at addressing structural shortcomings of EU's crisis response and long-standing problems for which member states have been unable or unwilling to find a solution. The creation of a European Health Union (including specific measures to enhance health protection of EU citizens, to equip the EU and member states, to prevent and address future pandemics, to improve resilience of member states' health systems, to revise the mandate of the ECDC and EMA and to create a new EU agency for biomedical preparedness), the reinforcement of coordination and information sharing (interoperability) of the structures responsible for crisis management at the EU and member state levels, the reform of the Schengen area, the proposal for a new EU own-resources system and the emphasis on the social dimension of the economy are examples of envisaged changes that resulted from (or were revived because of) the lessons of the pandemic.

Some of the Commission's proposals are ambitious enough for a truly transformative change. Most likely, however, in the course of the negotiations for their adoption the ambition will be toned down by the need to accommodate member states' different preferences and visions, resulting at best in boosted incremental change. Yet, the integration process is moving forward. COVID-19 crisis was an important reminder that cooperation fosters solutions that represent a win for all the players, whereas egoistic strategies normally end up in zero-sum (or even negative sum) games. Ultimately, the deepening of European integration as a result of the management of the pandemic crisis will only be feasible if member states continue to endorse common responses to common problems (even when confronted with asymmetric problems and payoffs). This would most likely entail accepting and promoting a more prominent role for the EU in several policy areas, including crisis management and, maybe, health policy. Hence, the potential for the development of European integration ('more Europe', as it is currently labelled) is to be confirmed by future events.

Notes

1 The terms 'affective' and 'utilitarian' support were used by Leon N. Lindberg and Stuart A. Scheingold in their seminal work *Europe's Would-be Polity* to mean, respectively, support that 'seems to indicate a diffuse and perhaps emotional response to some of the vague ideals embodied in the notion of European unity' and 'support based on some perceived and relatively concrete interest' (Lindberg and Scheingold, 1970, p. 40). The expressions draw on David Easton's (1975) diffuse and specific support.

2 Politico. 'Merkel: EU "Probably" Needs Treaty Changes, Especially for Health Policy'. 21 April 2021. Available online at: www.politico.eu/article/angela-merkel-coronavirus-europe-treaty-changes-health-policy/ [Accessed 26 April 2021].
3 The expression was used by the High Representative Josep Borrel in a statement addressing the COVID-19 pandemic on 24 March 2020. See EEAS. 'Delegation of the EU to China. EU HRVP Josep Borrell: The Coronavirus Pandemic and the New World It Is Creating.' Available at: https://eeas.europa.eu/delegations/china/76401/eu-hrvp-josep-borrell-coronavirus-pandemic-and-new-world-it-creating_en [Accessed 1 April 2021].
4 The use of strategic foresight in support of EU policymaking was first developed under Delors' *Cellule de Prospective,* but the Commission intends to mainstream it into policymaking in all fields (European Commission, 2020). In 2020 the Commission published its first Foresight Report.

Bibliography

Borrel, J., 2021. My Visit to Moscow and the Future of EU–Russia Relations, HP/VP Blog, 7 February 2021. Available at: https://eeas.europa.eu/headquarters/headquarters-homepage/92722/my-visit-moscow-and-future-eu-russia-relations_en. [Accessed 6 January 2020].

Easton, D., 1975. A Re-assessment of the Concept of Political Support. *British Journal of Political Science*, 5, pp. 435–57.

European Commission, 2020. *2020 Strategic Foresight Report – Charting the Course Towards a More Resilient Europe*. Available at: https://ec.europa.eu/info/sites/info/files/strategic_foresight_report_2020_1.pdf. [Accessed 27 November 2020].

Lindberg, L. and Scheingold, S. 1970. *Europe's Would-be Polity: Patterns of Change in the European Community*. Englewood Cliffs, NJ: Prentice-Hall.

Rhinard, M., 2019. The Crisification of Policy-making in the European Union. *Journal of Common Market Studies*, 57(3), pp. 616–33.

Streeck, W. and Thelen, K., 2005. Introduction: Institutional Change in Advanced Political Economies. In W. Streeck and K. Thelen, ed. *Beyond Continuity: Institutional Change in Advanced Political Economies*. Oxford: Oxford University Press, pp. 3–39.

Index

Note: Page numbers in **bold** refer to Tables